Coping with Hearing Loss and Hearing Aids

Debra A. Shimon, MS, CCC–A
Audiologist

SINGULAR PUBLISHING GROUP, INC.
SAN DIEGO, CALIFORNIA

For Bob, Betty, Dick,
Cindy, Jessica, and Jay

Published by Singular Publishing Group, Inc.
4284 41st Street
San Diego, California 92105

© **1992 by Singular Publishing Group, Inc.**

Typeset in 11/14 Times by CFW Graphics
Printed in the United States of America by McNaughton & Gunn

Library of Congress Cataloging-in-Publication Data
Available on Request

ISBN 1-879105-45-4

❖ Table of Contents

❖ Foreword

The books in the *Coping with Aging Series* are written for men and women coping with the challenges of aging, and for their families and other caregivers. The authors are all experienced practitioners: doctors, nurses, social workers, psychologists, pharmacists, nutritionists, audiologists, physical and occupational therapists, and speech-language pathologists.

The topics of individual volumes are as varied as are the challenges that aging brings. These include: hearing loss, low vision, depression, sexual dysfunction, immobility, intellectual impairment, language impairment, speech impairment, swallowing impairment, death and dying, bowel and bladder incontinence, stress of caregiving, giving up independence, medications, and stroke. The volumes themselves, however, share common features. Foremost, they are practical, jargon-free, and responsible. Each contains professionally valid information translated into language people who are not health care providers can understand. Each contains useful advice and sections to help readers decide how they are doing and whether they need to do more, do less, or do something different. Each includes lists of services, suppliers, and additional readings. Each provides evidence that no single person need cope alone.

None of the volumes can substitute for appropriate professional health care. However, when combined with the care, instruction, and counseling that health care providers supply, they make coping with aging easier.

America is greying at the same time its treasury is inadequate to meet its population's needs. Thus the *Coping with Aging Series* offers help for people who need and want to help themselves.

This volume, *Coping with Hearing Loss and Hearing Aids,* is written by a professional audiologist with twelve years of experience in hearing loss and in the fitting of hearing aids. If you, or someone you know, is considering a hearing aid, this book will help. If you have a hearing aid but are dissatisfied, this book will tell you what can be done. If you want to know more about hearing, aging, or what can be done for you or someone you care about, this book will give you answers in words you can understand. No person who has a hearing loss needs to be isolated in a world of silence.

John C. Rosenbek, Ph.D.
Series Editor

Molly Carnes, M.D.
Medical Editor

❖ Preface

Presbycusis, or hearing loss from aging, is one of the most common disorders of growing older. An estimated 16.4 million Americans have hearing loss, and at least one third of them are 65 years of age or older. Hearing loss has been called the "silent" handicap because it can't be seen and because it is not widely recognized by society as a problem. Approximately 10 million people with presbycusis have not sought professional hearing help or have not followed the professional advice they received when they did. This means that a great number of Americans are needlessly enduring the hardships created by hearing loss. If you are one of those millions of Americans, or if you care for one of them, you will find this book useful.

Hearing help is easily accessible and is available to you, to family members, and to friends. Hearing health care professionals can competently diagnose your hearing problem and recommend the appropriate course of action.

Approximately 1.4 million hearing aids are sold each year, and much of the revenue is used by manufacturers to develop better and better hearing aids to give you the best possible hearing. To get the most benefit from hearing aids, however, it is important for you to understand how they work and what they can and can't do. And, it is critical for you to be fitted with the hearing aids that are best for your hearing loss.

Coping with Hearing Loss and Hearing Aids is written for people with hearing loss and for their families, friends, and caregivers. It provides a thorough explanation of hearing health care professionals, the ear, hearing loss, and the effect hearing loss has on communication. Chapters to help you cope with your hearing problems and to improve your communication, both with and without hearing aids, will increase your confidence in social situations. Hearing aids are demystified, and current hearing aid technology is explained. Included is a two-week program designed to get you started wearing your new hearing aids as well as complete information about using them effectively and caring for them. Hearing aid repair information and troubleshooting their malfunctions at home are also covered.

Finally, there is a resource chapter which lists organizations you may contact for further information about hearing loss, hearing devices, and hearing help. The list includes companies from which you may order products made specifically for people with hearing loss.

Special thanks are accorded to Russ Rohrdanz and Beth Larimer for reading the manuscript and for offering professional recommendations.

Chapter 1

Recognizing When You Have a Hearing Loss

Presbycusis (prĕz-bĭ-kū′-sĭs) means hearing loss from aging. It is a common problem, affecting at least 30% of those 65 years of age and older. In fact, it is eight times more common in people 65 years and older than in those 45 years of age. Different people have different amounts of hearing loss from aging, and the extent to which hearing loss worsens over time also varies from person to person. Presbycusis is not life threatening and it is not painful, so you do not need to worry that your health is affected by it, but it may interfere with your enjoyment of conversation and of people in general.

Presbycusis can be an inconvenience to you and to those who are close to you. There are some tell-tale signs of hearing loss which you may recognize in yourself and which others may recognize in you. This chapter is designed to help you, and the people close to you, discover if you have some hearing loss.

Signs of a Mild Hearing Loss

The term "mild" may be misleading because it implies that there isn't much of a problem, but if you have such a loss, it can be quite significant. Hearing loss, even a mild one, makes conversation sound soft and like the person speaking is mumbling. Some of the problems you may notice if you have a mild loss are listed below. You may notice all of them or only a few, and they may be more pronounced in some situations than others.

1. You can hear people talking but you can't understand them easily, especially when more than two or three people are talking.

2. You can hear people talking but you can't understand them easily when there is background noise.

3. You have difficulty hearing and understanding people when they are more than 10 feet away from you.

4. You have difficulty hearing dialogue on TV and at movies, and you turn the TV volume higher than others prefer.

5. You watch people closely when they talk and understand them better when they face you.

6. You accuse people of not enunciating properly.

7. You guess at what people have said and pretend to have understood them when you haven't.

8. You monopolize a conversation so you know what is being discussed.

9. Attending social activities leaves you tired and out of sorts.

10. You withdraw from social activities.

Some of the things others may notice in you or things they may have to do to communicate with you if you have a mild hearing loss are listed below. These are listed because many people with hearing loss do not realize that people close to them know about the hearing loss and may be doing things to make communication easier.

1. They may frequently repeat or rephrase what they say.

2. They may have to talk louder and turn the TV louder when they are with you.

3. They think you don't pay attention to them when they talk to you and may even accuse you of this.

4. They may "translate" the conversation of others so you know what was said.

5. They may notice that you talk louder than normal.

6. They may notice your speech is changing. You may slur some words or drop word endings, like a final "s" sound.

7. They may hear you make an inappropriate comment because you have misunderstood the conversation.

8. They may notice you withdraw from social activities.

Signs of a More Severe Hearing Loss

Hearing loss may, or may not, progress beyond the "mild" classification. If it does, the communication problems you have will increase as well. Some of the signs of a more severe hearing loss are listed below. You may notice all of them or only one or two.

1. You can hardly hear or understand people talking most of the time.

2. People must be facing you when they talk or you don't understand any of what they are saying.

3. You ask for most things to be repeated.

4. You avoid social activities and feel left out when you do attend because you can't hear what is being said or you feel ignored.

5. You try to explain your hearing problem away. You find yourself saying or thinking that most people don't say anything worth listening to anyway, or that you are not interested in what they are saying so it doesn't matter if you don't hear them.

If you have a more severe hearing loss, your hearing problem will be obvious to the people who live with you or care for you. It will cause both you and those people great inconvenience and anxiety. If they choose to keep trying to communicate with you, they will have to do several things:

1. They will have to repeat most things they say to you.

2. They will have to talk much louder than normal.

3. They will find that communication works best when they face you and stay within 3 to 6 feet of you.

4. They may sometimes not talk to you because the effort it requires is so great.

If you, or those around you, recognize some of these signs and want to do something about them, help is available. You and they do not need to be adversely affected by a hearing problem. If you suspect that you have a hearing problem based on the signs in this chapter, your next step should be to seek an evaluation of your hearing and recommendations for hearing help from a hearing health care professional. Chapter 2 will guide you in the selection of such a person.

Chapter 2

Hearing Health Care Professionals

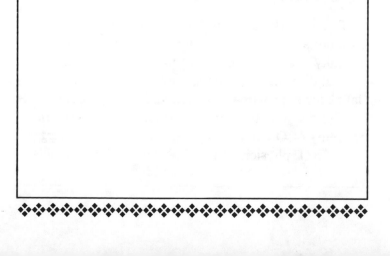

Hearing health care professionals determine whether or not you have a hearing loss, how much of a loss you have, and what you can do about it. They are the people you should turn to for answers to your questions about hearing. It is important to find the best services available for your hearing needs. Three types of hearing health care professionals are available and you may see one, two, or all three of them at one time or another, in any order.

1. Ear-Nose-Throat (ENT) Physician

2. Audiologist

3. Hearing Aid Specialist

This chapter describes each profession, the services each can offer you, and the qualifications required to practice each of them. The Food and Drug Administration (FDA) regulations that hearing aid dispensers must meet before selling a hearing aid are also found in this chapter. Finally, suggestions for finding reputable hearing health care services are offered.

Ear-Nose-Throat (ENT) Physician

ENTs are physicians who are also referred to as otologists, otolaryngologists, or otorhinolaryngologists. Their specialty is the diagnosis and treatment (including surgery) of diseases of the ears, nose, and throat. They specialize for approximately 5 years after completing medical school and are board certified by the American Academy of Otolaryngology—Head and Neck Surgery. Some ENT physicians also specialize in facial plastic surgery. In addition to this national certification, physicians are licensed by the state(s) in which they practice.

What the ENT Physician Does for You

The ENT physician can determine whether your hearing loss is treatable with medication or surgery based on a visual examination of your ears and a complete hearing evaluation. In some cases, additional tests, such as special x-rays and scans, may be needed for the ENT physician to rule out ear, nerve, or brain diseases that can cause hearing loss, headaches, ear ringing (tinnitus), imbalance, and dizziness or vertigo. He or she will also check the general health of your ears. The ENT physician plays a vital role in ensuring there are no serious medical causes of your hearing loss and in providing treatment when necessary.

The ENT physician takes a history of your ear and hearing problems and visually examines your ears with an otoscope (medical flashlight with an ear tip or cone) or a specialized microscope. The ear examination the ENT physician performs may seem quick to you, but in that inspection, he or she can determine if your ear canals and eardrums appear normal. The ENT removes excess ear wax only if there is any to remove. Wax can result in a slight hearing problem, but it is usually not the total cause of your hearing loss.

After the examination of your ears and the hearing evaluation (see Chapter 3) are completed, the ENT physician will talk to you about the type and extent of your hearing loss. If medication is required or if surgery is an option, he or she will discuss that with you. If there is no medical treatment for your hearing loss, a hearing aid probably will be recommended. Most ENT physicians do not test hearing or dispense hearing aids themselves. Approximately 70% of them employ audiologists for these purposes.

Audiologist

Audiologists (ŏ-dī-ŏl'-o-gĭsts) are trained in the measurement and diagnosis of hearing disorders and the rehabilitation of communication problems caused by these disorders. They have a graduate college degree (Master's or Ph.D.) and the Certificate of Clinical Competence in Audiology (CCC-A) awarded by the American Speech-Language and Hearing Association. Audiologists are licensed in 39 states. In addition, audiologists in many states are also licensed as hearing aid/instrument dispensers. Audiologists may work in universities, hospitals, with speech-language pathologists/therapists or ENT physicians, or in their own private practices.

What the Audiologist Does for You

The audiologist administers a complete hearing evaluation to determine if hearing loss is present, how much is present, and what type of hearing loss you have. The hearing evaluation is described in Chapter 3. The audiologist will either interpret the test results for you or will provide the information to the ENT physician. In medical settings, hearing loss is considered to be a medical diagnosis, and the information about your loss may be delivered by the physician.

Audiologists are communication and hearing instrument specialists. Therefore, if your hearing loss is not medically treatable by the ENT physician, the audiologist can recommend communication treatment for you. This treatment may include: counseling about your hearing loss, ways to improve communication, and hearing aids. Usually, the audiologist is also a hearing aid dispenser and you can purchase an instrument from him or her. Audiologists who dispense hearing aids also provide servicing of them. If the audiologist does not dispense hearing aids, you will be provided with a list of reputable hearing aid dispensers in your area. Some audiologists, especially those in university departments, also provide speechreading (lip reading) instruction and other lessons to improve your communication skills and help you to cope with hearing loss. More information about these techniques is found in Chapter 6.

Hearing Aid Specialist

Hearing aid specialists, also referred to as hearing aid dealers or hearing instrument specialists, are business and sales people who sell and service hearing aids. They are trained in the measurement of hearing and hearing aid dispensing but university study is not required. An apprenticeship with a practicing hearing aid specialist usually is required as is passing a licensing exam in most states and the District of Columbia. Only Colorado and Massachusetts have no regulatory board overseeing hearing aid specialists. In addition, some hearing aid specialists are certified by the National Board for Certification of Hearing Instrument Sciences (BC-HIS). The National Hearing Aid Society (NHAS), which oversees this licensing board, requires that specialists attend continuing education seminars and pass a national examination for certification. Hearing aid specialists may no longer call themselves "Hearing Aid Audiologists" because this title may mislead you into thinking you are seeing an audiologist when you are not.

What The Hearing Aid Specialist Does For You

Hearing aid specialists are trained to do limited hearing testing and recommend hearing aids. Although their educational requirements are less comprehensive and technical than an audiologist's, many possess a great deal of knowledge and practical experience. It is estimated that hearing aid specialists fit over half of the hearing aids sold in this country. They often travel to people's homes and to nursing homes to provide services. In rural and remote areas, they may provide the only services available for hearing help. Hearing aid specialists also provide hearing aid servicing.

Scheduling an Appointment with the Hearing Health Care Professional

You may feel confused about which hearing health care professional to see first. The reason is because there is no single "right" or "wrong" way to proceed when seeking information about your hearing loss. Because it is important to be sure that there are no health problems that could be causing your hearing loss, the appointment order should be scheduled as follows:

1. ENT physician — to rule out medical problems with your ears.

2. Audiologist — for a complete hearing evaluation.

3. Audiologist or Hearing Aid Specialist — to obtain hearing aids if needed.

This order of seeking hearing help complies with the Food and Drug Administration's requirements for adequate hearing health care before obtaining a hearing aid.

Food and Drug Administration Hearing Aid Regulation

The Food and Drug Administration (FDA) enacted a regulation in 1977 which requires that certain conditions be met in the hearing aid delivery system. "Dispenser" is the FDA term for any person who sells hearing aids and includes ENT physicians, audiologists, and hearing aid specialists. The term *dispenser* is used from here on to refer to anyone who sells hearing aids. A summary of the FDA regulation follows:

1. Dispensers must advise you to consult promptly with a physician (preferably an ENT specialist) before dispensing a hearing aid if you have certain symptoms of

ear disease, such as drainage, pain, sudden hearing loss, or conductive hearing loss (see Chapter 4).

2. Dispensers must have a signed statement from your physician (preferably an ENT physician) which declares that your ears and hearing were medically evaluated and that you are considered a candidate for a hearing aid. This exam must be current within 6 months.

3. You may waive the medical examination, but the dispenser must advise you that this is not in the best interest of your health.

4. Dispensers cannot encourage you to waive the medical examination.

5. Dispensers must obtain your signature on the waiver.

6. Dispensers must advise patients who have a hearing condition to consult with a physician.

The FDA requirements just listed are the minimum guidelines that dispensers in all states must follow. State licensing boards may impose further restrictions on the testing of hearing and the dispensing of hearing aids. For example, in Wisconsin, no waiver is permitted or accepted for a person under 18 years of age, and the hearing test for any individual must be current within 6 months. All children must be seen by a physician prior to being fitted with hearing aids. If your hearing is tested in a medical clinic or hospital, you may find in your state that you will not be offered the option of waiving the medical examination of your ears. If you go to a hearing aid specialist for hearing health care services, he or she must advise you to see a physician, and if you decline, he or she must have you sign the waiver.

Finding a Hearing Health Care Professional

People select a specific hearing health care professional in a number of ways. You may feel most comfortable asking your family physician for a recommendation or asking a friend who has a hearing loss or wears a hearing aid for a recommendation. Local senior citizen centers and coalitions often have listings of health services available in your area. Your regular medical clinic or hospital may also have an ENT physician and/or audiology department. Many people consult the Yellow Pages of the telephone book to find services near their homes. The categories in the telephone book to look under are:

1. ENT physicians or otolaryngologists

2. Audiologists

3. Hearing aids

4. Hearing

Finally, you may call professional organizations for the names of professionals in your area. The addresses and descriptions of each organization are found in Chapter 14.

1. American Academy of Otolaryngology
   (703) 836-4444

2. American Speech-Language-Hearing Association
   Helpline for Consumers
   (800) 638-8255

3. National Hearing Aid Society
   Hearing Aid Helpline
   (800) 521-5247

Finding Reputable Hearing Health Care Services

Hearing health care and selling hearing aids are big businesses. You may be aware of hearing aid sales abuses, deceptive advertising, and professional competency issues reported in newspapers and magazines. If you have any doubts about a hearing health care professional, or if you'd just like to be sure about the individual you select, there are ways to find out if he or she has ever been reported.

All states have a medical licensing board for physicians and most states have licensing boards for audiologists and hearing aid specialists. These boards keep records of members who have had complaints issued against them and whether or not any action was taken. You may call these state departments and ask about your hearing health care provider. A complete list of state regulatory agencies for Hearing Aid Specialists and licensing agencies for Audiologists is provided on pages 193 and 199 in Appendices A and B.

You can call the toll-free Doctor Certification Line at (800) 776-2878 to find a physician who has been certified by the American Board of Medical Specialties, for which specialty, and in what year.

The state Attorney General's Office and the Better Business Bureau in cities are also sources for the same information. Look for the numbers in your telephone book.

All of these services exist, in part, for consumer protection. If you have a serious problem with your hearing health care professional, you may file a complaint yourself. It is a help to all consumers when people take action against poor hearing health care.

Your Hearing Health Care Professional

You can rest assured that help for your hearing problem exists. Hearing health care professionals are there to be of service and to meet your hearing and ear care needs. They are a knowledgeable and competent group of professionals who are trained to provide you with optimal hearing help. Do not hesitate to avail yourself of their services. They want you to hear better, too!

Chapter 3

The Hearing Evaluation

The hearing evaluation is a battery of tests, not just one test. Its purpose is to determine how much hearing loss you have, whether you have hearing loss in one or both ears, and which parts of your ears are causing the hearing loss. Your ability to hear and understand speech is also tested. This chapter begins by describing hearing screenings, which are not hearing evaluations, but simply procedures that tell you whether or not your hearing is normal. The chapter goes on to describe the tests given in a complete hearing evaluation, the test equipment that is used, and the cost. It is important for you to know what to expect when you go to the hearing health care professional for testing.

Hearing Screenings

If you are reluctant to pursue a hearing evaluation, an easy way to begin finding out about your hearing problem is to go to a hearing screening sponsored by a medical clinic, hospital, health fair, hearing aid specialist, or senior citizens' center. Announcements of hearing screenings are usually posted in the senior citizens' events section of local newspapers or in senior citizens' centers. In some areas, medical clinics and hospitals sponsor a free telephone hearing screening that you can call from your home. Call 800-222-EARS (or 800-345-EARS in Pennsylvania) for the free telephone hearing screening number in your area.

The purpose of a screening for any disorder (for example, hearing, vision, blood pressure, glaucoma) is to identify whether or not a problem exists. You either "pass" or "fail" a screening; that is, either there is a problem (fail) or there isn't (pass). A screening does not necessarily tell you how much of a problem, in this case hearing loss, is present or what kind of a hearing loss it is. The screening just tells you that your hearing is not normal.

You should be given a summary of the screening results (pass or fail) and recommendations to seek further testing if you fail. You may be referred to your family physician for further instruction. If you go to a hearing aid specialist for a hearing screening, it may be recommended you set up an appointment for more complete testing at that office. If you fail any hearing screening given anywhere, a complete hearing evaluation by an audiologist and an ear check by a physician are recommended in Chapter 2 as the most appropriate way to find out more about your hearing.

A hearing screening should *never* be viewed as a complete evaluation, and no one should attempt to sell you a hearing aid based on such a rudimentary test. A hearing screening is simply one way to begin. It also is an easy way for family members or caregivers to get you to realize your hearing is not as good as it used to be. A screening doesn't usually require an appointment or a fee. It may be the ideal way to get you, or any other person, to think about hearing loss and communication.

The Hearing Evaluation

The hearing evaluation is made up of several tests aimed at discovering your hearing acuity for the low-, middle-, and high-pitched sounds (tones) that comprise speech and at how well you hear and understand speech. Important tests that provide information about the workings of your middle and inner ears and your hearing nerve are also administered. A hearing evaluation is accomplished with specialized equipment in a quiet environment, preferably a soundproofed room.

The Test Equipment

Hearing testing is done with an audiometer (ŏ-dī-ŏm-ĕ-ter). An audiometer produces different pure-tone frequencies (pitches) at varying intensities (loudnesses). The tester can present tones of different pitches from very soft to very loud. The audiometer also has a microphone and/or a tape deck or compact disk player so that the tester can either speak to you or present recorded speech to you at varying intensities.

The tones and speech the audiometer presents are heard through headphones (earphones) placed over your ears. Tones are also presented through a bone conduction vibrator, a headband device, which is placed on the mastoid bone behind your ear. The picture on the facing page shows a person's hearing being tested through earphones with an audiometer.

The Hearing Test Environment

Hearing testing should be conducted in a soundproofed booth, as shown in the picture, so that background noise does not complicate test results. Exceptions to this are for

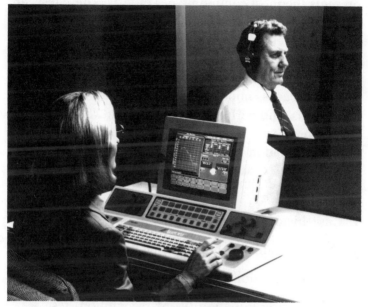

Courtesy of Nicolet Instruments Corporation

**Hearing testing in a sound-proofed booth using an
audiometer with headphones**

home-bound or hospitalized patients and for special testing done in factories. Hearing testing should not be done
in your home (unless you are home-bound), stores, shopping malls, or hotel rooms. During testing, you should be
turned away or isolated from the tester so that you can't
see him or her present tones and speech.

The Hearing Evaluation Test Battery

Hearing health care professionals do not all administer
the same tests or use the same test materials. This section

presents the most common types of tests. These tests are the minimum to expect as part of your hearing evaluation. They represent thorough testing which leads to a more accurate diagnosis of hearing impairment and thus the most appropriate treatment. Correct interpretation of tests is at least as important as administration of the tests themselves, and perhaps more important. The better the tester's professional training, the better the testing and the interpretation of the test results.

The hearing evaluation usually includes the following:

1. Case history

2. Pure-tone air and bone conduction tests

3. Speech reception test

4. Speech discrimination (word recognition) test

5. Acoustic immittance test

6. Most comfortable listening level and uncomfortable listening level assessment.

Each of these is described in the following sections.

Case History

The audiologist (or hearing aid specialist) will ask you or you should be sure to volunteer the following information:

1. What you perceive to be your hearing problem.

2. How long you have noticed a hearing problem.

3. If your hearing is poorer in one ear than the other or if they seem to be the same.

4. If your hearing problem came on suddenly or gradually and if you've noticed changes in your hearing recently.

5. Whether anyone in your family (including parents and grandparents) has had a hearing problem.

6. If you experience pain or drainage from your ears or if you get wax build-up frequently.

7. If your ears ring or if you have head noises.

8. If you have episodes of dizziness, spinning, imbalance or falling.

9. If you have had ear surgery or if your ears have been injured.

10. If you have worked around or with noisy machinery (for example, in construction trades, factories, farming, aircraft, guns) either recently or in the past.

Before testing begins, you will be ushered into a sound-proofed booth or room. You will sit in a comfortable chair and be instructed about what to listen for and how to respond. Be sure to ask for clarification if something doesn't make sense to you. Testing usually begins with earphones being placed on your ears.

Pure-Tone Air and Bone Conduction Tests

These are tests administered with the audiometer presenting different pure-tone frequencies (pitches) at different intensities (loudnesses). The tones sound like low-, mid-, and high-pitched beeps. Each ear is tested separately through both the earphones (air conduction) and the bone conduction vibrator (bone conduction). The two methods of testing indicate whether the hearing loss is in the middle ear or in the inner ear and nerve (see Chapter 4).

You are asked to signal each time you hear a tone, usually by raising your hand or pressing a button. You should signal even when the tones are so soft you can barely hear them. The tester increases and decreases the loudness of each tone to find the level at which you can just barely hear it. The softest level at which you can hear each tone is called your pure-tone threshold. Thresholds are plotted on a graph called an audiogram.

The Audiogram

Your hearing impairment is measured by the loudness in decibels (dB) of hearing level (HL) for each pure tone. The decibel scale is like a thermometer. The higher the temperature, the greater the number of degrees. The greater the hearing impairment, the greater the loudness of the tone and the greater the number of decibels.

Pure-tone pitches are designated in Hertz (Hz). Low pitches have a lower Hertz number, and as the pitch of the tone gets higher, the Hertz number gets larger. A low-pitched tone, 250 Hz, roughly corresponds to the pitch of traffic noise. A high-pitched tone, 8000 Hz, roughly corresponds to higher notes played on a flute. The pure tones between 250 and 8000 Hz are chosen for testing because speech encompasses these frequencies or pitches.

The audiogram (ŏ-di-ō-grăm) is a graph of the loudness (in dB) of the threshold (the softest level you hear a tone) for each pure-tone frequency (pitch) that is tested. Different symbols depict hearing for each ear for air and bone conduction tone presentation. An audiogram is shown on the next page.

The audiogram is arranged with frequency (pitch) in Hz across the top line, from low to high pitches (250-8000 Hz), and intensity (loudness) in dB along the side, from very soft to very loud (-10 to 110 dB). If you hear the frequency 1000 Hz at 50 dB, for example, a mark is made on the audiogram where the lines intersect.

Hearing loss is classified by hearing level, or extent of hearing loss, according to the decibel scale as follows:

Normal hearing	-10 to 25 dB
Mild hearing loss	25 to 40 dB
Moderate hearing loss	40 to 55 dB
Moderate to severe hearing loss	55 to 70 dB
Severe hearing loss	70 to 90 dB
Profound hearing loss	>90 dB

Speech Reception and Discrimination Tests

The speech reception test is designed to measure the softest level at which you can just hear and understand words. Two-syllable words (for example: baseball, mush-

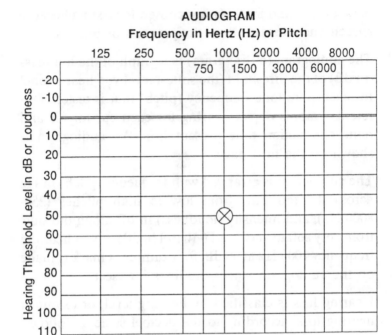

AUDIOGRAM
Frequency in Hertz (Hz) or Pitch

X = Left Ear
O = Right Ear

An audiogram is used to plot the softest level (threshold) at which you can hear low-, mid-, and high-pitched tones in each ear. A 50 dB threshold is marked at 1000 Hz (a mid-pitched tone) for both ears as an example.

room, sidewalk) are presented through earphones, and you are asked to repeat them. If you have difficulty speaking, you are asked to point to pictures or to write the words. The tester increases and decreases the loudness of the words to find your threshold for speech reception.

The speech discrimination (word recognition) test is a measure of how accurately each of your ears (and sometimes both ears together) is able to distinguish speech sounds in words. One-syllable words (for example: wood, all, bill) are presented through earphones at a constant, comfortable loudness, and you are asked to repeat them (or point to or write them). Twenty-five or 50 words are presented to each ear individually (and sometimes to both together). A score of percent correct is computed and your speech discrimination is classified as excellent, good, fair, or poor. This test usually is given in quiet but sometimes, background noise is added to simulate more difficult listening situations.

Acoustic Immittance Tests

Acoustic immittance testing involves two procedures that give the hearing health care professional information about the workings of your eardrums, middle ear bones, and the hearing nerve. These parts of your ear are described in Chapter 4.

The tests are called tympanometry (tĭm-păn-ŏm´-ĕ-trē) and acoustic reflex testing. Both are accomplished by putting a small plug in your ear while you sit quietly. The plug fits tightly, but is not uncomfortable. You do not have to make any responses for these tests. They are done quickly on each ear. You feel a brief air pressure change (tympanometry) and then you hear some loud tones (acoustic reflex testing). The tones are not painfully loud, but they may startle you or be unpleasant if you are sensitive to loud sounds. These tones last only 1 to 10 seconds each.

Comfortable and Uncomfortable Loudness Levels

If the tester determines that hearing aids could be useful to you, these additional measures are incorporated into the test battery. These levels can be established using pure tones, speech, or both. As the test names imply, these are the loudness levels (in dB) at which you find speech (or tones) to be the most comfortable to listen to and the point at which they become uncomfortably loud in each ear. It is important to determine how much a hearing aid should amplify sound so that it is comfortable to you and to make sure that sound is not amplified to an uncomfortably loud level.

The preceding sections covered the basic testing that you can expect as part of your hearing evaluation. Other tests are done once you actually have a hearing aid. These tests are described in Chapter 12.

Results of the Hearing Evaluation

After the hearing evaluation is completed, the hearing health care professional will explain the results to you. You will be told the extent (mild, moderate, severe) of your hearing loss and how well you hear and understand speech in each ear. The implications of your hearing loss on your daily communication will be discussed. You will also be told if your hearing loss is permanent or if it can be treated with medication or surgery. If hearing aids can help you, they will be discussed in detail. As always, if you have questions about the test, the results, or the recommendations, you should feel free to ask for clarification. It is very important for you to understand as much as possible about your hearing.

The Cost of a Hearing Evaluation

Hearing evaluations are not inexpensive. In 1992, complete evaluations cost approximately $110.00 at medical clinics and usually more at the office of a private practice audiologist. The physician's examination of your ears is an additional cost. Some hearing aid specialists include the cost of the evaluation in the price of the hearing aid. However, since nothing is ever really free, their hearing aids usually cost more than those obtained at medical clinics and hospitals. When you schedule your appointment, you should ask how much the testing will cost and whether the cost of testing is separate from the hearing aid charge. You can call several places and compare costs. Many insurance plans, Medicare, and Medical Assistance (Title XIX) cover at least a portion of the doctor's examination and the hearing testing. Hearing aids are *not* covered by most insurances or by Medicare.

Chapter 4

The Ear
And Hearing Loss

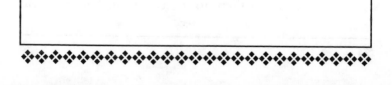

We depend on all of our senses to stay in contact with the world around us. Hearing is considered the most important sense by many, and the ear is the intricate mechanism that permits this sense to function. The ear has thousands of moving parts and is, thus, extremely complex. The ear and hearing mechanism described in this chapter are duplicated on each side of your head. This chapter provides an overview of the structures and common disorders of the ears. Hearing loss associated with problems in each part of the ear, including those from aging, is discussed.

For your general understanding, only a few common disorders of the ears are covered in this chapter. This information is not for self-diagnosis of ear disease. Anytime you experience ear symptoms such as pain, drainage, hearing loss, ringing or buzzing sounds, dizziness, or imbalance, you should consult your physician.

Knowing about the ear and the hearing mechanism leads to a better understanding of your own hearing loss and which parts of your ears are affected. You will also understand why some hearing and ear problems can be treated by the physician and some can't. This ultimately helps you make the decision of whether or not you need a hearing aid.

The ear is discussed as a three-part system: the outer ear, the middle ear, and the inner ear and nerve.

The Outer Ear

The purpose of the outer, or external, ear is to collect sounds and funnel them to the eardrum. The outer ear (see illustration below) has two parts: the pinna or auricle and the ear canal.

The Pinna

The pinna, or auricle, is the outermost part of your ear, that is, the part attached to your head which is commonly called the "ear." It is made of skin-covered cartilage and is the least important part of the ear for hearing. People without a pinna are able to hear as long as the rest of the ear is formed normally. The pinna's shape has developed to emphasize sounds important for hearing speech. The pinna changes with aging and becomes larger. The lobe

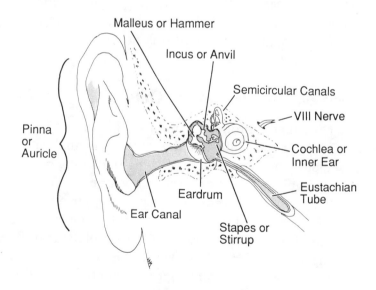

Cross section of a right ear

may elongate and, in men, bristly hairs may sprout from it and from the ear canal.

The Ear Canal

The ear canal is the channel leading from the pinna to the ear drum and is about 1 inch long in adults. It is what the hearing health care professional looks into when examining your ears. The ear canal has two types of glands which excrete substances. When the substances combine, ear wax, or cerumen, is formed. Small hairs keep ear wax moving toward the outside of the canal. This action helps keep them clean and keeps foreign objects (for example: insects or dirt) from getting farther inside the ear. Different people produce different amounts of ear wax, so there is no "normal" amount. Whatever amount you produce is normal for you.

Common Disorders of the Outer Ear

The ear canal is prone to wax blockage. To clean your ears each day, wipe the opening of the ear canal with a washcloth, but do not stick anything (including bobbie pins, toothpicks, or cotton swabs) in your ears. The saying "Never stick anything smaller than your elbow in your ear" is true and should be observed. You may injure the skin of the ear canal washing it with solutions or by gouging it with sharp objects. You also may push the wax farther in or even puncture your eardrum by attempting to clean it yourself. If your ear canals are blocked with wax, have it removed by a physician.

Another common problem of the ear canal is an infection called external otitis. This is often called "swimmer's ear," but it can develop when the ear canal is moist from any reason, not just from swimming. This condition may itch or be painful, and the ear canal may feel wet. External otitis requires treatment by a physician.

If any liquid or sticky substance ever drains from your ear canal, consult your physician as soon as possible. This may indicate an infection in the ear canal or middle ear that requires medical treatment.

The Middle Ear

The purpose of the middle ear (see illustration on page 35) is to transmit sound from the outer ear to the inner ear. This may seem simple but it requires converting sound waves from the ear canal into vibrations of the eardrum and a chain of three bones to the inner ear fluid. The middle ear is an air-filled space and contains the following parts:

1. The eardrum or tympanic membrane

2. Three middle ear bones or ossicles

3. Eustachian tube

The Eardrum

The eardrum, or tympanic membrane, is a semi-transparent, pearly-gray colored membrane. It is what is seen at the end of the ear canal when the hearing health care professional looks into your ears. It forms the physical border between the outer and middle ears. This membrane vibrates when sound from the ear canal impinges on it.

Disorders of the Eardrum

The eardrum can develop a hole, which is also called a perforation. Common causes of perforation are trauma to the head (for example: being hit) and ear infections. Perforation can result when fluid produced by an ear infection causes the eardrum to burst. They often heal by themselves once the infection is treated. Ear infections do not always cause perforations. Some adults, however, have continuous ear infections which can result in a persistent perforation. The ENT physician can evaluate whether or not this perforation can be surgically repaired.

When the physician examines your ears, he or she checks the color and appearance of your eardrums. In cases of infection, they may appear dull or red, and fluid may be seen behind them. In cases of perforation, a small hole can be seen.

The Middle Ear Bones

Collectively, the three bones of the middle ear are called the ossicles, or ossicular chain, and they are the smallest bones in the body. The bones are called the malleus (hammer), incus (anvil), and stapes (stirrup) and are shown in the illustration on page 35. They attach to the eardrum at one end and to the inner ear at the other end. The vibration of the eardrum is transmitted along the ossicular chain to a membrane covering the inner ear, thus setting inner ear fluid in motion. The middle ear cavity in which these bones sit is air-filled.

Disorders of the Middle Ear Bones

Probably the most common disorder of the middle ear bones is otosclerosis (ō-tō-sklĕ-rō′-sis) or a hardening of the bones in the ear. Otosclerosis is caused by extra bone growth over the existing bones and the joints between them. It may occur in one or both ears and is most common in Caucasian women. It is a progressive disorder, meaning it usually worsens with time.

The new bone growth in otosclerosis causes the bones to fixate and not vibrate efficiently, so sound does not pass through the ossicular chain as well. The result is a hearing loss. The ENT physician may be able to operate and free the fixation or replace the stapes with a prosthetic, man-made device. If surgical treatment is not possible or if it does not work, a hearing aid may be recommended.

Less commonly, these bones can become disconnected from a blow to the head or ears or from repeated, severe ear infections. When this happens, sound vibration along the chain is disrupted and hearing loss results. The ENT physician may be able to reattach the bones or substitute a prosthetic, man-made device in place of the affected bone(s). If treatment fails or is not possible, a hearing aid may be recommended.

The Eustachian Tube and Middle Ear Space

The eustachian tube (see the illustration on page 35) passes from the middle ear space to the back of the throat where the nose and throat join. It cannot be seen by looking in the ear or throat. Its function is to equalize pressure in the middle ear space. The eustachian tube is usually closed but it opens during yawning, sneezing, swallowing, and vigorous nose blowing. You probably have experienced the pressure equalizing effects of this tube when ascending or descending in an airplane or even when driving in the mountains. Your ears feel plugged, so you swallow and then your ears pop open. This "popping" results from the eustachian tubes opening to equalize pressure.

Disorders of the Eustachian Tube and Middle Ear Space

Colds and sinus and throat infections can affect the eustachian tubes. They may be unable to open and close properly as a result. The tissue lining the tubes can become inflamed causing the feeling of stuffy ears. If the cold and tissue swelling goes away, you may hear and feel a pop or crackling in your ears, signifying that the eustachian tubes are beginnning to function normally again. The stuffy feeling disappears and your hearing returns to the way it was before the cold.

In some cases, however, the tubes do not reopen, and the pressure in the ears causes the tissue lining to secrete fluid. The middle ear space then fills with fluid, and your hearing becomes poorer. This condition is called a middle ear infection and requires treatment by a physician. Ear infections can be quite painful. If not treated in time, fluid can burst through the eardrum and drain out of the ear canal. Untreated ear infections can lead to other, more serious infections. Do not treat yourself by using hot compresses on the ear or warmed oil in the ear. See a physician.

Other diseases can cause the ears to feel plugged but do not involve the eustachian tubes. Do not diagnose yourself. Consult your physician when you experience plugged ears and/or decreased hearing.

Conductive Hearing Loss and the Outer and Middle Ears

The hearing loss caused by disorders of the outer and middle ears is called a conductive hearing loss. The name is logical. The disorders described in the previous sections result in disruption or blockage of sound conduction through the ear. An estimated 5 to 10% of all hearing losses are conductive.

Conductive hearing loss usually goes away if the condition causing it can be treated medically or surgically. When the wax is removed or the ear infection and fluid clear up, for example, so does the conductive hearing loss. Surgery on the eardrum and middle ear bones is the most common form of surgery. In some cases, medical treatment is not possible or does not completely reverse the conductive hearing loss. In these cases, a hearing aid can be useful.

The Inner Ear and Nerve

The purpose of the inner ear (see the illustration on page 35) is to convert the vibrations delivered from the middle ear into a form of energy that stimulates the hearing nerve to send nerve impulses, or information, to the brain, resulting in hearing. The inner ear also functions as the body's balance system. The inner ear cannot be seen by looking in the ear. It is located inside of and is protected by the skull.

Hearing Function of the Inner Ear and Nerve

The hearing portion of the inner ear is also called the cochlea (kōk-lē-ah). It is a winding, snail-shaped, pea-sized structure with three main chambers. Within these chambers are thousands of specialized cells called hair cells. The hair cells are bathed in special fluids. The movement of this fluid causes the hair cells to bend in response to the vibrations from the middle ear bones. It is this bending action of the hair cells that activates the nerve cells connected to them. The combined activation, or firing, of nerve cells sends impulses along the hearing nerve to the brain. The hearing nerve is called the auditory nerve and is a branch of cranial nerve VIII. Your brain interprets these impulses as sound, and it is your brain that actually "hears."

Balance Function of the Inner Ear

The balance portion of the inner ear is called the labyrinth or vestibule. Attached to the cochlea via a small channel are three ring-shaped, fluid-filled canals called the semicircular canals (see the illustration on page 35). These canals contain specialized cells that move and bend in response to your head's movement. The semicircular canals are arranged perpendicularly to each other to correspond to all positions of your body. Simply put, when the canal is stimulated by head movement it tells the body its position and helps keep proper balance. The specialized cells in the semicircular canals activate the nerve cells attached to them. An impulse is sent along the balance, or vestibular, nerve to the brain. The vestibular nerve is also a branch of cranial nerve VIII.

Disorders of the Inner Ear

Disorders of the inner ear involve damage to or disintegration of the hair cells and problems with vestibular system. Because the hearing and balance systems are connected, disorders sometimes affect both your hearing and your balance. This section primarily covers disorders affecting hearing, but includes a description of Meniere's disease, which is both a hearing and balance disorder.

The hair cells of the cochlea can wear out or be destroyed by a variety of causes. Common causes of disintegration are aging, excessive noise exposure, diseases (for example, meningitis, diabetes), some medications (for example, streptomycin, vancomycin, cis-platin), head injury, and heredity. Presbycusis, or hearing loss from aging, is most often a combination of hair cells wearing out, noise exposure, and heredity.

When hair cells are worn out or damaged, they do not regenerate. The effect of the damage of the cells is to cause hearing loss. The nerve cells connected to the hair cells may also lose function and they do not regenerate either. Therefore, damage to these structures is permanent. In addition to hearing loss, you also may experience ear ringing or head noises, but no pain. Usually, but not always, both of your ears will be affected to the same degree. A surgically implanted device called a cochlear implant may be useful for the most severe forms of deafness, but it does not restore hearing.

Meniere's Disease

Meniere's (mĕn-ē-ār′-z) disease, named after the physician who reported it, is a disorder involving both the balance and hearing systems of the inner ear. It develops from abnormal fluid pressure in the vestibular portion of the inner ear, which then increases pressure on the hair cells in the cochlea. It usually starts with one ear but may affect both ears over a period of years. The symptoms typically are a feeling of fullness or pressure in the ears, a roaring sound in the ears, and progressive hearing loss in the affected ear. Other symptoms include sudden attacks of vertigo (spinning, whirling sensations), which can be quite severe, nausea, and imbalance. The hearing loss may become worse during these attacks. Proper diagnosis of this disease should be made by your physician. Treatment may involve medication, surgery, or both. A hearing aid often is used in addition to the medical treatment.

Sensorineural Hearing Loss and the Inner Ear and Nerve

Hearing loss resulting from disorders of the inner ear and/or hearing nerve is called sensorineural (sensory-neural). The hearing loss is usually a combination of damage in the inner ear (sensory) and the nerve (neural). This loss is commonly referred to as "nerve loss." Such a loss is usually permanent and can continue to worsen. The hearing loss usually is not treatable by medication or surgery, even if the disorders causing the hearing loss are. Once the hair cells are damaged, there is no way to replace them or make them whole again. Sensorineural hearing loss is not painful and can't be seen by looking in the ears. It is the most common type of hearing loss, accounting for about 90% of all hearing losses. Most people who wear hearing aids have "nerve," or sensorineural, hearing loss.

The hearing loss that develops from aging, presbycusis, is a sensorineural hearing loss. Further information about presbycusis is found in the next chapter.

Mixed Hearing Loss

It is possible to have both a conductive and a sensorineural hearing loss at the same time. This is called a mixed hearing loss. You may have a sensorineural loss from aging and also get an additional conductive loss, for example, from ear wax. Removing the ear wax relieves the conductive part of the hearing loss but does not improve the hearing loss from aging.

This chapter described the ear and the hearing loss that results from problems in different parts of the ears. The next chapter explains the effect that hearing loss has on communication.

Chapter 5

The Effect of Presbycusis and Other Factors on Communication

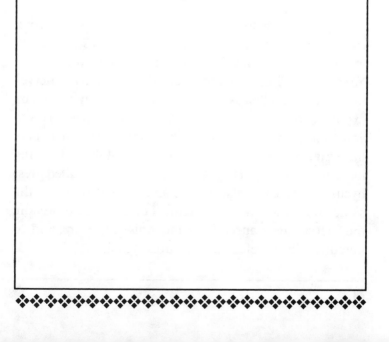

The way you hear and understand people talking is influenced by several factors. Presbycusis is the major factor, and the greater the extent of your hearing loss, the greater the communication difficulties you experience. Your general health makes a difference too. If you are not well or if you have memory problems, for example, your ability to concentrate and listen may be compromised. Also, environmental factors such as background noise and distance from the person speaking have an important effect on how you hear and understand others.

This chapter explains the influences of the amount or extent of hearing loss and environmental factors on communication, with an emphasis on the effect of hearing loss from aging, or presbycusis.

How Presbycusis Affects Communication

Presbycusis, or hearing loss from aging, causes some specific effects on communication. Other causes of hearing loss besides presbycusis may cause similar difficulties. Your hearing loss may have been diagnosed as a "nerve" loss. Your hearing loss may have been partially caused by exposure to loud noises or it may have been passed on to you from previous family generations. Presbycusis may have many causes. Aging is simply one of them. Hearing loss caused by any of the above factors may be called presbycusis, if you are also aging, and all will result in the same communication problems. For ease of discussion, the "nerve" loss caused by aging, noise exposure, and/or heredity will be referred to as presbycusis.

Presbycusis does not get better, but it can get worse over the years. Because it results from changes (for example, deterioration) in the inner ear and hearing nerve, it is considered a permanent, sensorineural ("nerve") hearing loss, and there is no medication or surgery to improve it. Hearing loss from aging is not painful, and it cannot be seen by looking in the ears. It affects all of us to differing extents.

Presbycusis typically affects hearing in the high pitches to a greater extent than hearing in the low pitches. This doesn't necessarily mean you will have more trouble hearing women than men, but this is a common complaint. Women usually speak more softly than men, and it is the softer voice which causes the difficulty rather than the pitch of the voice. However, a hearing loss for high pitches will cause difficulty hearing the chirping of birds, although you will probably hear the low-pitched sound of a train, even at a distance.

Another noticeable effect is that your voice may be louder than normal. Because you have a hearing loss, you need to talk loud enough to hear yourself and to overcome your hearing loss. Your voice won't seem loud to you; it will sound just right. But other people will notice that you speak loudly.

Presbycusis not only makes speech sound soft but it also affects the clarity of words so that people may sound like they're mumbling. Presbycusis can be simulated by tuning a radio station so that it is not properly tuned in but sounds distorted, or unclear, and then turning the volume down. It is difficult to hear the radio station, and it is also difficult to understand what is being said. You can turn the volume back up so that it is easier to hear, but the clarity of the words will still be poor. Usually, people with presbycusis need both volume and clarity to improve how they hear people talking. Hearing aid selection requires considerable skill because inappropriate hearing aids can make communication worse or even be physically uncomfortable, especially if too much volume is provided.

"I Can Hear You But I Can't Understand You"

This familiar phrase is frequently expressed by people with presbycusis. You probably have even said it yourself in various situations. Hearing people talking but not understanding what they are saying is caused by the typical hearing loss from presbycusis, which is greater for higher pitches than for lower pitches. This may not seem to make much sense but this section explains how clarity and high pitched hearing loss interact.

The audiogram, or hearing graph on the facing page, shows the average amount of hearing loss for people of different ages, from 40 to 80 years old. It illustrates the progression of hearing loss with increasing age and also demonstrates that hearing for the low pitches is less affected than hearing for the high pitches, regardless of age.

Now turn to page 52 and look at the illustration that shows where different environmental and speech sounds are plotted on the audiogram. This picture shows the pitches and loudnesses at which some speech sounds occur in conversation. In general, conversational loud-

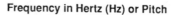

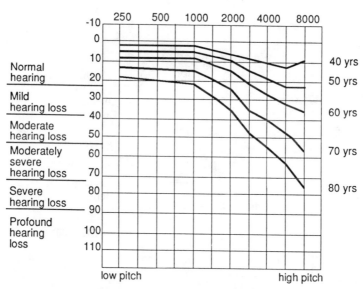

Adapted from U.S. Army Environmental Hygiene Pamphlet (1980)

Progression of high frequency hearing loss with aging

ness is between 40 and 50 dB, but individual sounds are made up of different pitches. Vowel sounds, such as *a, i, o, u,* and *e* are found on the left, or low-pitched, side of the graph at 40 dB. Some consonant sounds such as *s, f,* and *th* are on the right, or high-pitched, side of the graph at about 20 dB. This means that vowel sounds tend to be lower in pitch and louder than consonant sounds, which tend to be higher in pitch and softer. If you have a high-frequency (pitch) hearing loss, you will hear vowels better, in general, than you will hear consonants. Consonant sounds are more numerous than vowel sounds in our

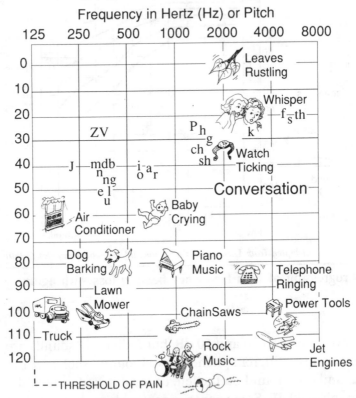

Adapted from **Hearing in Children** *(4th ed.) by J. L. Northern &*
M. P. Downs, 1991. Baltimore, MD: Williams & Wilkins.

Common speech and environmental sounds shown on an audiogram

language so words are more frequently differentiated by consonants. For example, the words *sin, fin* and *thin* all have the same vowel. The consonants make them different words. Not hearing consonant sounds well makes speech sound less clear and it is more difficult to distinguish, or discriminate, words. This is what the speech discrimination test described in Chapter 3 measures.

Simply increasing the volume of the words won't necessarily improve your speech discrimination ability. The volume of the higher pitched sounds needs to be increased to a greater extent than the volume of the lower pitched sounds. This is what hearing aids try to do.

Effects of the Extent of Hearing Loss on Communication

The extent to which you have presbycusis affects communication and causes predictable difficulties hearing and understanding people talking. The effects of hearing loss on communication are organized according to the amount, or extent, of your hearing loss in the chart on the next page. Refer to Chapter 3 to review decibels (dB) and the measurement of hearing loss.

To put the numbers on the chart in perspective, softly rustling leaves are about 0 to 10 dB while a whisper is about 20 to 30 dB. Normal conversational loudness at a distance of 3 feet is about 45 to 50 dB. The sound of a baby crying is about 60 dB. Heavy traffic or a person shouting is about 90 dB. And a jet's engines are far greater than 110 dB. These and other sounds are plotted on the audiogram

Effects of Severity of Hearing Loss on Communication

Severity of Hearing Loss	Classification	Effects on Communication
0–25 dB	Normal	None or slight
25–40 dB	Mild	Conversation sounds soft and muffled. Could benefit from a hearing aid.
40–55 dB	Moderate	Conversation sounds very soft or is barely heard. Hearing aid is needed.
55–90 dB	Moderate-to-severe and severe	Can't hear conversation. Must use hearing aid to hear conversation.
>90 dB	Profound	Difficulty hearing conversation even with a hearing aid.

on page 52. If you have a moderate hearing loss of approximately 50 dB, for example, you will not hear leaves rustling, and a baby crying would sound very soft. Conversation would be only faintly audible.

The classification of hearing loss by the categories mild, moderate, moderate to severe, severe, and profound is convenient. However, it is not only possible, but common, to have different amounts of hearing loss at different pitches. You may have a mild hearing loss for some pitches and a severe hearing loss for other pitches.

The classification system also assumes equal hearing loss in each ear. It is possible to have hearing loss only in one ear or to have hearing loss that is worse in one ear than the other. When your hearing is better in one ear than the other, the classification system describes the effect on communication based on the hearing in your better ear. Hearing loss in only one ear causes an additional communication problem. It is difficult, or impossible, to tell where sounds are coming from because they always sound as if they are on your better side. Equal hearing in both ears is required to be able to localize or tell the direction of a sound.

Extent of hearing loss can be a hard concept to grasp. This is because there are no common references in daily life to equate with a "mild" or a "moderate" hearing loss. Instead, people usually ask what the percentage of their hearing loss is.

Percentage of Hearing Loss?

Percentage of hearing loss probably makes intuitive sense to you. It seems logical that if you have a 30% hearing loss, then you've lost one third of your hearing and have two thirds left. There is even a formula to figure out a hearing loss percentage, and some hearing health care professionals still use it. However, hearing and hearing loss are misrepresented by a percentage figure, because a percentage does not take into account that you can have different amounts of hearing loss at different pitches. Instead, it averages the extent of your hearing loss across several pitches. It is possible to compute a 30% hearing loss by the formula if you have, for example, about a 35 dB hearing loss for all pitches: low, middle, and high. But you could also compute a 30% hearing loss if you have normal hearing for low pitches and a moderate or severe hearing loss for high pitches. The percentage is the same, but the hearing loss is very different.

Even though it may seem cumbersome to describe your hearing loss by categories (mild, moderate, severe), it is the most accurate way to do so. And since it is most common to have different hearing at different pitches, it is best to describe your hearing loss by pitch range; for example, a mild hearing loss for low pitches and a moderate loss for high pitches.

Other Factors that Influence Communication

The type and extent of your hearing loss are the primary factors in your ability to hear and understand people talking, but environmental factors such as competing background noise and reverberation and the distance you are from the person speaking are important too. These factors are further explained in the following sections.

Background Noise and Reverberation

Regardless of the amount of hearing loss you have, you may have noticed that you hear and understand conversation better in a quiet room than in a noisy one. You also may have noticed that it is easier to talk with one person at a time than to converse in a group of people. This too can be blamed on presbycusis, a hearing loss which is greater for higher than for lower pitches.

Background sound or noise is primarily low in pitch and may be relatively loud compared to conversation. This is true of television noise, restaurant noise, and the noise associated with people talking in the background. If you have presbycusis, your hearing is probably better for low pitches than for high pitches, so you can easily hear the the low-pitched background noise. The noise covers up or drowns out the higher pitched consonant sounds that you may have some trouble distinguishing even in quiet surroundings. In addition, reverberation of noise from hard walls, ceilings, and floors further degrades the conversation you are trying to follow. Conversation may be *heard* through this background noise, but it will be difficult to *understand.*

People with normal hearing also experience difficulty following conversations in noisy places; hearing loss makes it even more difficult.

Distance from the Speaker

It is intuitively apparent that the farther away you are from the person speaking, the more difficult it is to hear what is being said. In fact, the person's voice becomes twice as soft with the square of the distance. That means the speaker will sound twice as soft at 9 feet away as when you are only 3 feet away. That decrease in loudness may be enough so that you can't hear what he or she is saying if you have even a mild hearing loss. Optimal communication distance is 3 to 6 feet from the person you are talking with.

This chapter described some of the detrimental effects of presbycusis, the extent of hearing loss, and environmental factors on your ability to communicate. Some important ways to positively influence your communication and to cope with hearing loss are covered in the next chapter.

Chapter 6

Ways to Improve Communication

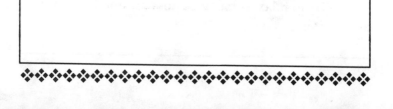

Improving your communication involves some common-sense actions. This chapter is designed to encourage you to think about what interferes with your hearing and understanding, and it provides you with suggestions to improve or overcome communication difficulties. You can implement many of them quite easily without anyone even knowing you are doing so. Speechreading (lip reading) is one strategy and it is covered in detail. This chapter applies to you whether or not you have hearing aids or intend to get them. Hearing aids can amplify the sounds you are missing but they do not replace good communication practices. There is also a section with suggestions for family members and caregivers to improve communication with you. The chapter begins by relating good communication practices with accepting your hearing loss. Acceptance is actually the first step toward improved communication.

Accepting Your Hearing Loss

You can greatly improve your ability to understand people by relaxing, having a sense of humor, and accepting that you have a hearing problem. Relaxing can keep you from panicking when you temporarily lose the thread of conversation. It is impossible for anyone to hear and understand every single word another person says when there is some background noise or in groups of people. Don't put pressure on yourself to keep up with every sentence in a conversation, but don't give up on participating either. Try to relax as much as possible and listen as well as you can.

Having a sense of humor is useful because sometimes you are going to make a mistake about what you think you heard. If you can laugh a little and take it in stride, you won't be so embarrassed and neither will those you are talking with.

Being able to do those things, though, depends on your acceptance of your hearing loss. Accepting your hearing loss may be difficult or it may be easy for you. It depends on your personality, your attitudes about hearing loss, and how you perceive yourself. Most of your friends and family members will be aware that you have a hearing problem, so if you can admit it also, there will be no need for you or others to pretend it doesn't exist. Try using phrases like:

"I have a hearing problem,

  would you please repeat?"

  would you face me please?"

  would you slow down please?"

Try these phrases first on family members and close friends. Practice saying "I have a hearing loss" to others and to yourself. It won't make people think less of you or reject you, and many will try to be more accommodating when you don't understand what they've said.

The following sections provide strategies to help you overcome difficult communication situations and to improve your everyday conversations.

Strategies For Better Communication

If you have a hearing loss, you are well aware that it is more difficult to hear, and especially to understand, someone talking when there is noise in the background or if you are conversing in a group of people. It is also difficult to hear a person who is across the room from you. This section addresses these difficult communication situations and provides strategies to overcome or improve them. The strategies to improve these factors are:

1. Improving your communication environment

2. Improving your communication by using visual communication cues; that is, by speechreading

Improving Your Communication Environment

In the previous chapter you learned that background noise, reverberation, and distance from the speaker interfere with your hearing and understanding by covering up speech sounds (especially consonants) and by making the speaker's voice softer. Since these two factors seriously compromise how you communicate with a person, it is to your advantage to improve the environment as much as you can. These common-sense suggestions should be implemented whenever possible.

Keep Background Noise to a Minimum

1. Turn off the TV, radio, or stereo when you are talking with other people. Background music may create a nice setting, but it interferes with communication.

2. Move to a different spot in the room if you are near an air conditioner, fan, or other noise source as these create background interference.

3. At a restaurant or meeting, ask to be seated at a table away from large groups, preferably in a corner, to reduce noise on one or two sides of your table.

4. In a setting where tables are in rows, sit at the end table to reduce surrounding noise.

5. Entertain in small groups of people rather than large groups. There will be less interference from people talking to each other. You may also enjoy yourself more in a small group because it is easier to follow the conversation.

6. If you have a choice, always select a quiet restaurant over a noisy one for easier communication.

7. Try to converse in rooms with carpeting and drapes or other sound-absorbing materials. These items reduce reverberation of noise. Conversation will be easier to follow if you avoid sitting near walls, windows, and other hard surfaces.

Reduce Your Distance from the Speaker

1. *Try to talk with other people only when they are in the same room with you.* This may require some effort on your part to go to the same room or ask that person to come to you. The effort is necessary to decrease frustration, however, because it is so difficult to hear what is said from a different room.

2. *Sit at the front of the church, temple, meeting room, or lecture hall.* Sitting at the back of a room means you will not hear the speaker at the front. Sitting at the front also allows you to watch the person who is talking. Some public places have speaker systems mounted on the walls. You can sit near one of these if you can hear and understand the person's voice comfortably.

3. *At a social gathering, try to sit or stand next to the person you want to talk with so you can hear him or her better.*

Improve Your Communication with Speechreading

You probably have noticed that you "hear" someone better when he or she faces you while speaking. Conversely, you may have noticed that you lose parts of the conversation when a person turns his or her back to you while still speaking. You may still hear the person talking but you may not understand what he or she was saying. This is because you have been speechreading.

It has long been known, both intuitively and from research studies, that watching a person talk improves how well you hear and understand. An older term for this is "lip reading," but this process involves more than just looking at a person's lips. When someone is speaking, you watch their facial expression; jaw, lip, and mouth movements; and you listen for the context of the conversation. Since this technique means you are aware of many aspects of communicating all at once, it is more broadly and more accurately called "speechreading."

Practicing this technique helps you make the most of a difficult listening situation and helps you set expectations for yourself. Speechreading helps in a great many, but not in all, situations. It is not true that you can understand everything a person says by watching his or her lips, regardless of what is portrayed in spy movies.

Knowing the benefits and limitations of speechreading helps you be an educated, more relaxed, and efficient communicator. These benefits and limitations are explained and some specific instructions for speechreading are provided in the next section.

Benefits of Speechreading

Speechreading makes you a more active, interested communicator by focusing your attention on the speaker(s) and the context of the conversation. This is done by:

1. Being visually observant and keeping your eyes on the speaker whenever possible.

2. Being an active listener by concentrating on the topic or context of the conversation.

3. Being an active participant in the conversation and asking for repetitions as needed.

4. Setting realistic expectations for yourself based on knowledge of what speechreading can and can't do.

Limitations of Speech Reading

Two very important limitations of speechreading are the result of characteristics of speech sounds, and they prevent you from speechreading every single sound in a word and every single word in a conversation.

1. *Some sounds and words look alike on the lips and mouth.* These are called *homophonous* (hō-mŏf-ĕn-ŭs) sounds and words. For example, the sounds *b, p,* and *m* are all made by putting the lips together the same way. Consider the words "ban," "pan," and "man." On the lips they look identical, but of course, they are completely different words. The context of the conversation can help you decide which of the words was actually said.

2. *Some sounds and words are invisible on the lips and mouth.* These sounds and words are called invisible because they are made entirely inside the mouth with little or no jaw, mouth, or lip movement. For example, the sounds *n, d, t, g, k,* and *ng* are invisible. It is even possible to say a whole sentence of invisible words. The familiar question, "It's a nice day, isn't it?" is invisible. Watch yourself say this in a mirror and you will barely see any movement of your mouth. You may hear a person speak these words, but it will be very difficult to speechread and you may miss some of the conversation.

Instructions for Speechreading

Speech flows, one sound into another and one word into the next. Because speech flows, speechreading does not involve concentrating on single sounds or even on single words. Learning to read this flow comes naturally. We all do it and rely on it somewhat, without thinking or formal instruction, whether our hearing is normal or impaired. Some of us are better at it than others, but everyone has some minimal skill in it.

If you don't believe you can speechread, try this demonstration. When you are with another person in a somewhat noisy setting, for example, a restaurant, just converse normally with that person. Then ask the person to hold the menu in front of his or her mouth and continue talking. You will notice right away that you have trouble understanding what is being said and you will have to concentrate very hard on the sound of the person's voice. You may not even be able to understand what that person is saying. Then ask your friend to lower the menu so you can watch him or her talk again. Right away, you will find it easier to follow the conversation. Understanding speech by listening and watching at the same time is speechreading.

These following techniques can help you sharpen your skills:

1. *Position yourself so you can see the speaker.* Ideally, you want to keep the speaker's face in the light so you can see it clearly. Try not to sit or stand so that the light is shining in your own eyes. Rather, position yourself with your back to the window or lamp. A lamp to the side of the speaker and indirect lighting also work well.

2. *Keep your eyes on the speaker's face.* In this way, you can continuously observe the speaker's mouth and facial

movements and expressions. Good eye/face contact makes you a more attentive listener with the added benefit that the speaker feels you are very interested in what he or she is saying.

3. *Listen for the context and key words and phrases rather than to each individual word.* You can't catch every single word in a conversation all of the time. Do not be alarmed when a word, phrase, sentence, or paragraph gets by you. Instead, keep the topic or context of the conversation in mind, so that certain key words or phrases can guide you back on track.

   For example, if you have been talking about stock market investments, you might expect to hear words like "stocks," "bonds," "interest," "Wall Street," or many others to occur. The context cues you into what you can expect to hear, and key words or phrases cue you into the specifics of what is being said. You don't need to understand each word to be able to participate in a conversation.

4. *Listen to the flow of the speaker's voice.* The inflection and flow of a person's voice signals when questions are asked by a rising voice inflection. The end of a sentence or thought is signaled by a pause. Important points are made by increasing voice loudness and emphasizing words. These cues can provide additional information about the conversation.

5. *Be aware that certain types of words and changes in the topic of conversation will be difficult to follow.* Proper names, dates, and numbers or a change in the topic of conversation are all unpredictable. The reason key

words and phrases keep you in the conversation is because they help you predict what is said. However, when a person introduces him- or herself or when a number or date is mentioned, you have no way to predict it. Likewise, when the topic of conversation changes, you have no way to predict what will come up next. It may take you several sentences to catch up.

6. *Ask for repetitions whenever you need them.* If you become confused, do not be afraid to ask for a repetition. You can do this in a variety of ways rather than just asking "what?" or "hunh?" Some examples are:

> "Would you please repeat that?"
>
> "I'm sorry, I missed what you said."
>
> "Pardon me?"
>
> "Did you say _____?"
>
> "Are you talking about _____?"
>
> "I have a hearing problem, would you please say that again?"

Other Factors that Influence Speechreading

A number of other factors influence your ability to speechread and can make it more difficult. Some of these you can influence but some you can't. Being aware of them helps you set your expectations for how speechreading works.

1. *The speaker talks too fast.* Ask him or her to speak more slowly. When someone talks too fast, it is more difficult to sort out the words.

2. *The speaker doesn't move his or her mouth much or mumbles.* You can ask the speaker to enunciate more carefully but speaking habits are very difficult to change and your suggestion may not be appreciated.

3. *The speaker exaggerates mouth movements.* This is what may happen when you tell someone not to mumble. Speech is always easiest to understand when a person just talks naturally and doesn't distort words.

4. *The speaker's face is obscured from your sight.* Some people have the habit of talking with their hands in front of their faces or of looking down or away. Ask such people to look at you or to move their hands if you feel comfortable doing so. Mustaches and beards also obscure mouth movements, and those men who have them may be harder to speechread.

5. *The speaker has a speech problem or an accent.* Speech problems and accents distort the way sounds are produced and the words may have a different sound and inflection. Foreign speakers are typically difficult to speechread.

6. *The speaker talks too loudly.* This also distorts the way sounds and words are produced and also distorts the voice. Again, ask the person to speak naturally.

7. *A group of people are conversing.* Group conversations are more difficult to speechread because the speaker is always changing. This requires you to find the next

speaker after he or she has begun talking. Conversation may trade off rapidly between group members, making it even harder to keep up. Furthermore, you can't face each person in the group as they speak so it is more difficult to maintain good visual contact. Follow the conversation visually as well as you can and listen for key words which clue you into the topic.

8. *The lighting is poor or you are visually impaired.* Good lighting and good vision help you see the speaker's face. In poorly lit places, like many restaurants, you will have more difficulty speechreading and following the conversation. If your vision is poor, you also will have greater difficulty speechreading. If you wear glasses, make sure your prescription is current and corrects your vision as optimally as possible.

9. *The speaker is too far away to see easily.* Distance affects not only your ability to hear, but also makes speechreading more difficult. Move closer whenever you can.

10. *You don't look at the speaker.* It should be obvious by now that you have to watch and listen to a person talk to improve your ability to hear and understand. Some people, however, do not look at people's faces, whether from habit or from thinking it's rude to do so. If you are one of these people, you need to practice watching others more closely or you will always have difficulty understanding them. Begin by practicing on friends or family members. It is difficult to change your communication habits, but it is possible.

Speechreading Lessons

Speechreading techniques can be taught, and classes are available. The lessons focus on the techniques mentioned in the above sections and on improving your listening skills. Improving your listening skills is called "auditory training." Lessons often begin in quiet settings with only one or two other speakers and move to progressively more difficult settings with background noise and multiple speakers.

Speechreading and auditory training are often given as group lessons. The group is generally small, perhaps 3 to 10 people. Group sessions offer you several benefits. You have the opportunity to meet other people who experience and understand your communication frustrations. This creates a supportive atmosphere for you to discuss your experiences and to problem-solve them as a group. It can be helpful to find out what strategies others use when they are having communication difficulties and it can be helpful for you to share your own strategies. A group setting gives you a chance to practice these strategies so that you can be comfortable with them when you need to use them outside of your lessons. Finally, group lessons give you a chance to practice speechreading in quiet and noise, with two or more people.

Speechreading and auditory training lessons have helped many people improve their skills and be more comfortable in difficult communication settings. If you are interested in such lessons, you need to find where they are given. The most likely places to contact are the Communicative Disorders (or Speech and Hearing Science) departments at universities or colleges and the Speech

Pathology or Audiology departments in hospitals and medical clinics. The Alexander Graham Bell Association maintains a list of people and places that give speechreading lessons in some areas of the country. The address and phone number of this association are in Chapter 14.

Helping Family Members and Caregivers Improve Their Communication with You

People who live with you or care for you can do some things to improve their communication with you. This section is appropriate for both you and them to read. You have probably already guessed what the suggestions are if you have read the preceding sections. These suggestions should be followed whenever possible, whether it is a quiet or noisy environment and even if only two of you are conversing.

1. *They should get your attention before saying their whole message.* You may have difficulty catching the first few words someone says if you aren't aware that something is going to be said, especially if you were concentrating on something else. If people around you say your name first and hesitate until they have your attention, you will more easily hear and understand the whole message.

2. *They need to face you when they are talking.*

3. *They should speak naturally.* Speaking too loudly or exaggerating mouth movements distorts words. You probably need clarity more than loudness anyway, especially if you wear a hearing aid.

4. *They should slow their speaking rate slightly.* This provides extra "processing" time for you to figure out what was said.

5. *They should rephrase what they've said rather than just repeating it if you do not understand.* Rephrasing gives a different combination of sounds and words on the speaker's mouth. Possibly too many invisible or homophonous sounds and words were used, making it difficult to understand what was said.

6. *They should try to be within 3 to 6 feet of you for optimal communication.* Hearing loss makes it very difficult for you to follow a conversation from another room, so it is best if you are in the same room and not too far apart. That way you can see and hear them talking easily.

Your life doesn't have to change because you have a hearing loss. You can do the things you always do and see the people you most enjoy. The compensation strategies suggested in this chapter can help you in a great many situations. In combination with hearing aids, these compensation strategies may work even better for you. The following chapters help you explore your need for hearing aids and help you understand how to select and use them.

Chapter 7

Common Hearing Aid Myths

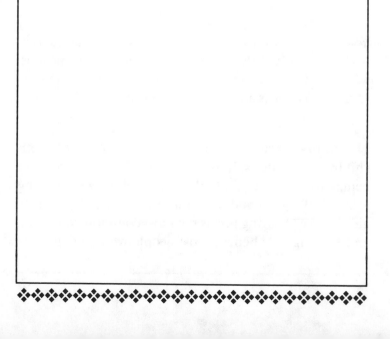

Before beginning a technical discussion of hearing aids, it is useful to counter any discouraging remarks you may have heard from other people about hearing aids. Common misrepresentations or myths about hearing aids could prevent you from even trying them. Myths are the result of misinformation, which may seem to make sense, but are founded on wrong premises. This brief chapter addresses five of the most common myths hearing health care professionals are questioned about by prospective hearing aid wearers. These myths need to be put to rest so you can approach hearing aids with confidence. You shouldn't deny yourself valuable hearing help because you've heard some incorrect information.

Myth 1: Hearing Aids Don't Help "Nerve Loss"

You may hear this from friends and physicians alike. This myth probably dates back to very early hearing aids, which had poorer sound quality, and to a time when ear surgery was not as advanced or as successful as it is today.

The truth is that most people who wear hearing aids, both children and adults, have "nerve loss." People who can benefit from ear surgery (only 5-10% of those with hearing loss) usually get it and do not necessarily need a hearing aid. "Nerve" hearing loss is the most common condition, and hearing aids benefit most people who have it.

Myth 2: Hearing Aids Change Your Hearing Loss

Hearing aids are man-made mechanical devices that have no curative powers. You will hear better only while wearing the hearing aids. When you take them off, you still have the same hearing loss. It will not have changed from having worn the hearing aids. Wearing hearing aids does not protect you from developing further hearing loss, nor does it cause more hearing loss. Research has suggested that not wearing hearing aids and, thereby, not stimulating your inner ears and hearing nerves, may eventually result in speech sounding less clear. However, either wearing or not wearing aids does not change your actual hearing loss.

Myth 3: Hearing Aids Cause "Lazy Ear"

Hearing aids do not have any effect on your ears that would cause them to quit functioning. If you only wear one hearing aid, your brain perceives sound to be coming only from that one ear. This is because sound is louder in the ear with the hearing aid and your brain pays attention to the most noticeable sound. However, this does not mean that the ear without a hearing aid no longer works or hears. It does. When you take the hearing aid off, you will have the same hearing you always do, in both ears. When you are wearing the hearing aid, it only seems that the other ear is not hearing.

Myth 4: Wearing Hearing Aids Makes You Dependent on Them

Hearing aids do not cause a physical or physiological dependence. You hear much better with your hearing aids on, and this makes listening easier and less stressful. When you take them off, the world is much quieter. You will feel less in touch with your surroundings, and you will have more difficulty hearing people talking. There is a big difference between hearing with hearing aids and hearing without them. You may interpret this to mean that you have become dependent on the hearing aids, but this is only true in the sense that you depend on them to hear better. You may forget how truly difficult it was for you to hear when you didn't wear hearing aids. This simply means that you have become accustomed to hearing with them and that you prefer wearing them to not wearing them.

Myth 5: Hearing Aids Don't Work Because I Know People Who Have Them and Never Wear Them

Adapting to hearing aids is different for every person. Most people are successful, but some are not. Another person's failure has nothing to do with you. You must try hearing aids yourself to know how they will work for you. Do not let someone else's experience discourage you from trying them.

It is unfortunate for any person to keep hearing aids in the drawer. Possibly that person doesn't really know how to use them or has unrealistic expectations. Perhaps the hearing aids are defective or are not appropriate for that person's hearing loss. There are many reasons why someone may not use his or her hearing aids; do not assume it's because they "don't work." If you know a person who has hearing aids but doesn't wear them, urge him or her to return to the dispenser or to make an appointment with an audiologist to have them tested. Perhaps a readjustment, or even different hearing aids, would allow that person to be a more successful hearing aid user.

You may hear these and other comments about hearing aids. Don't believe everything you hear. If you have a question about hearing aids, ask a professional hearing health care provider. Call your audiologist or hearing aid specialist rather than accepting the advice of an untrained person. Incorrect information, however well-meaning the source of it, promotes myths. Myths may keep people from getting the hearing help they need.

Chapter 8

Being a Good Consumer: What You Should Know Before Buying Hearing Aids

❖❖❖❖❖❖❖❖❖❖❖❖❖❖❖❖❖❖❖❖❖❖❖❖❖❖❖❖

If you have had a hearing evaluation and a doctor's examination of your ears and hearing aids have been recommended, some things are helpful to know and think about before signing on the dotted line. This chapter is designed to help you explore your need for hearing aids and your readiness to wear them. It is also intended to help you decide whether to buy one hearing aid or two. Included is a guideline of purchasing and service questions you should ask the hearing aid dispenser. This guideline also provides a way for you to compare services and policies of different hearing aid dispensers. You aren't simply buying a hearing aid off the shelf, you are actually purchasing a product with a host of services. To ensure you get a good hearing instrument and a good service provider, you are urged to be a good consumer by asking questions and shopping around. There's more to a hearing aid than its selling price.

Do You "Need" Hearing Aids?

Most people seeking hearing help ask the hearing health care professional whether or not they really "need" hearing aids. This can be a difficult question to answer because one person's definition of need is not the same as another's.

The question of need can partly be answered by the results of the hearing test. If you have even a mild hearing loss, you can be helped by hearing aids. The greater the amount of hearing loss you have, the more you need hearing aids. If you can barely hear people talking, you need hearing aids. But what if you hear well some times and have trouble hearing at other times? Does this mean you need hearing aids?

In general, if your hearing is troubling you enough to seek hearing testing and a hearing loss is diagnosed, you need hearing aids. The hearing health care professional will tell you if a hearing aid or aids can help you; true "need" is something you determine yourself. When you are ready to accept help for your hearing loss, you need hearing aids.

Being Ready to Wear Hearing Aids

You may examine your need for hearing aids, as described above, and conclude that you do need hearing help. That may not mean, however, that you feel ready to wear hearing aids. Hearing aids represent different things to different people. Some people embrace the idea of wearing hearing aids wholeheartedly and will take the necessary steps to hear better. Other people would like to hear better but not if it means wearing hearing aids. Some people know they have hearing loss but prefer their quiet world to remain as it is. Those who care about a person with hearing loss need to respect that person's right to decide whether or not to wear hearing aids.

Psychological readiness to wear hearing aids and motivation to make them work for you are very important factors in the success of your hearing aid experience. If you are being pressured by friends, family, or caregivers to get hearing aids but you don't want them, then perhaps you ought to wait awhile. You may need time to accept that you have a hearing loss and that hearing aids are the only way to improve it. You may also need time to realize that your hearing loss inconveniences you and those who care about you. It may be helpful to keep track of how often you:

1. Ask people to repeat.

2. Don't catch what someone says to you.

3. Get complaints from others about the volume of the television or that you're not paying attention.

4. Have an argument about your hearing.

If any or all of the above happen to you, then your hearing loss is affecting your life and the lives of those close to you. Very likely, your life would be easier and less stressful if you tried hearing aids, but you should be the one to make the decision.

One Versus Two Hearing Aids

Once you have decided to try a hearing aid, you have to decide if you will try an aid in one or both ears. Adults often wear only one hearing aid for economic reasons, not because they wouldn't hear better with two. In general, you will hear better with two hearing aids than one, just as you hear better with two ears than with one.

Sometimes the hearing test results will help you make the decision. If you have no hearing at all in one ear, your choices will be different than if you have equal hearing loss in both ears. You and the hearing aid dispenser should discuss if one or two hearing aids would be best, but you should make the final decision. Very likely, however, if you have hearing loss in both ears, the dispenser will recommend two hearing aids. Some considerations for choosing one or two hearing aids follow and may help you make the decision.

Choosing Two Hearing Aids

Here are some reasons for wearing two hearing aids for optimal hearing:

1. *You have hearing loss in both ears.* We have two ears for a reason: because our brains "hear" better in quiet and in noise with two ears. If you have hearing loss in both ears which is correctable with hearing aids, you should consider buying two hearing aids because you will hear better with two. Some research evidence suggests that if you only wear one hearing aid for many years, the ear without a hearing aid could lose some of its ability to distinguish speech sounds. Your inner ears and hearing nerves work best when they are stimulated with hearing aids in both ears. Remember, however, hearing aids don't cause you to have, or not have, more hearing loss.

2. *You are actively involved in life and in communicating with other people.* In this case, it is important for you to hear things equally on both sides. If you wear only one hearing aid, you will hear best on the side with the hearing aid. This can be a problem if, for example, you attend meetings or discussions where people are talking all around you, and you don't hear from both sides.

3. *You spend time in noisy places.* Research has shown that people hear better in noisy places with both ears working together, so you will hear better in noise with two hearing aids. Our brains cancel out a bit of noise and enhance speech when both ears hear equally.

4. *You feel "unbalanced" or "one-sided" by wearing only one hearing aid.* When you wear one hearing aid, you seem to hear only through the ear with the hearing aid. That can be an unnatural experience, and some people don't like it. It is also more difficult to hear people when they are talking on the side where you don't wear a hearing aid. If you presently wear one hearing aid and are not satisfied with it, you should consider wearing two.

5. *You can afford two hearing aids.* The price of two hearing aids may be double the cost of one. However, since your hearing is tested only once and both ears are tested, you should get a discount on the second hearing aid. If you have the resources to buy two hearing aids and the option to return one or both, you should consider trying two at the outset. Then you can decide if two are better than one during the trial period and make your own assessment of the benefits.

Choosing One Hearing Aid

If you have considered the reasons for wearing two hearing aids, but would prefer to start with one, you need to decide which ear to wear it in. It is not necessarily true that the hearing aid goes in the poorer ear, even though that may seem to make sense. Again, the hearing test results and the hearing aid dispenser may guide your decision.

Your hearing aid dispenser may suggest the following based on the hearing test results:

1. *Wear the hearing aid in the poorer ear.* You may wear the hearing aid in the poorer ear if the hearing in that ear can be improved enough to affect positively your overall hearing and communication. In some cases the poorer ear can be improved to the level of your better ear, which may be sufficient.

2. *Wear the hearing aid in the better ear.* You may wear the aid in your better ear if your poorer ear is so impaired that the hearing cannot be adequately improved with a hearing aid. This may be the case if you have a severe or profound hearing loss in the poorer ear but only a mild or moderate loss in the better ear.

3. *Wear the hearing aid in the ear with the best speech discrimination, if the hearing loss in both ears is equal.* The hearing evaluation will determine each ear's ability to discriminate, or distinguish, between speech sounds and words. If one of your ears has a better natural ability to understand words than the other, you should wear the hearing aid in that ear. However, having unequal speech discrimination between ears, with one ear being much better than the other, should not deter you from trying two aids. Very often two hearing aids are still better than one, even if one ear doesn't understand speech as well as the other.

If your hearing loss and speech discrimination are equal in both ears, it really doesn't matter which ear you wear a hearing aid in. Then you and the dispenser may consider some practical reasons for choosing one ear over the other based on your lifestyle:

1. *Handedness.* It may be physically easier and more natural to use your dominant hand to insert and manipulate the hearing aid. Some people also feel they have a dominant ear, just as they have a dominant hand.

2. *Telephone use.* If you hear well on the telephone and prefer to use one ear over the other, consider putting the hearing aid in the opposite ear. Most right-handed people use their left ears on the telephone, leaving their right hands free to write. The opposite is true of left-handed people. Telephones can make hearing aids squeal unless they are equipped with a special telephone switch (see Chapter 9). A hearing aid without a telephone switch may make phone use inconvenient. You can purchase or rent a telephone amplifier from the phone company. Chapter 11 explains how to use a telephone with different hearing aids, and Chapter 14 provides the names of different companies from which you can purchase telephone amplifiers.

3. *Car use.* If you spend a fair amount of time in a car and if you are usually the driver, consider putting the hearing aid in your right ear. That way, the hearing aid is toward your passenger and the radio and not toward the window where it will pick up wind and traffic noise. Conversely, if you are usually the passenger, consider putting the hearing aid in the left ear for the same reasons.

If none of the above are important considerations for you, simply pick the ear of your choice!

Consumer Guideline
For Purchasing Hearing Aids

Hearing aids are a major purchase and you should know the terms of purchase *before* you agree to them. Once you have signed a purchase agreement or contract with a hearing aid dispenser, it may be difficult to get out of it. You can save yourself a lot of time, trouble, and money if you find out the details of your purchase before you make it. Do not be pressured into a purchase, making a down payment, or signing a contract if you are not ready to do so or if you do not understand all the details. It may be helpful to have a family member or other support person with you for this discussion, especially it you are afraid you won't hear or understand all the details.

It is in your best interest to get the following information in writing before you enter into a hearing aid purchase:

1. *Cost of the hearing evaluation.* Ask if the test cost is included in the price of the hearing aids. If it is not, you should expect a separate bill and you should ask how much the charge is. Also ask if you can get a copy of the test results in case you want to get a second opinion. The cost of the ENT physician's ear exam is usually a separate charge from the cost of the hearing evaluation.

2. *Cost of the hearing aid or aids.* Ask for a written quote of the price and the terms of purchase before you pay. Also ask if you get a price break on a second hearing aid. Hearing aid price may vary by the style and the special

features it includes (see Chapter 9). If the hearing evaluation is a separate charge, the total cost is really the sum of numbers 1 and 2. Be sure to take all charges into account if you are comparison shopping.

3. *Hearing aid brand and model and the time it takes for the hearing aids to be delivered to you.* Ask the dispenser which brand and model of hearing aid he or she is ordering for you and how that decision was reached. Some dispensers sell only one brand; others carry several. If you have that information, you can comparison shop. It also provides you with the dispenser's rationale for choosing hearing aids. You will also need to know how much time you can expect to elapse between ordering the hearing aids and their delivery to you. Two weeks is reasonable.

4. *Trial period.* The FDA used to require hearing aid dispensers to provide a trial period for hearing aid use, but that is no longer a law. However, many hearing aid dispensers still offer a trial period (typically one month) in which you can return the hearing aids, but you should not assume you are getting one.

If a trial period is offered, ask what the cost is if you decide to return the aid. Trial periods are not necessarily free and you may forfeit some of the money you paid if you return the hearing aid. Some dispensers even charge you more for the hearing aid if you want a trial period. If you decide to try two hearing aids, find out how much is non-refundable if you return just one of them. Ask for this information in writing as part of the price quote.

You should further inquire about changing the style of the hearing aid or the ear you wear it in during the trial period and whether or not that costs extra. You may choose to try a different hearing aid or to switch it to the other ear, and you should know beforehand if that influences the trial period or the costs.

Finally, be sure that if there should be a problem with the hearing aids or if you should try different hearing aids, that you are still entitled to wear them for the full number of days specifed. Hearing aid manufacturing or fitting problems should not be allowed to use up your trial period.

5. *Payment for the hearing aids.* Be sure you understand when you have to pay for the hearing aids and whether you can make payments or are required to pay in full. Some dispensers require a down payment when you order the hearing aids, some require you to pay in full when you get them, and others require payment by the end of the trial period. Do not pay the full amount for the hearing aids *before* you get them. If you do not like a particular dispenser's payment policy, shop around.

6. *Follow-up visits.* Ask how many follow-up visits you are entitled to with the cost of the hearing aids and be sure you don't have to pay extra for problems that need attention during the trial period. Ask if hearing testing while wearing the hearing aids is included with follow-up visits. It is important to be sure the hearing aids are effective for your hearing loss.

7. *Hearing aid warranty.* Hearing aid manufacturers must provide the dispenser with a one-year warranty on a hearing aid according to FDA regulation. This means that the dispenser must pass that one-year warranty on to

the consumer. The warranty covers defects in workmanship and normal wear and tear malfunctions, but does not include accessories such as earmolds, batteries, or tubing (see Chapter 9). A warranty does not have to cover abuse from improper care. Some manufacturers also offer replacement of some hearing aids for a given amount of time, if they are lost, stolen, or damaged. Ask the dispenser how long the warranty is; if it can be extended; if loss, theft, and damage are covered; and if the warranty is included in the cost of the hearing aid. You will find that most dispensers do not charge extra for the warranty.

The warranty that comes with a hearing aid is not the same thing as an insurance policy. The warranty does not necessarily include loss or theft (though some do). If you are interested in hearing aid insurance, ask your homeowner's insurance agent if this can be added to your existing insurance (usually for an extra fee) or ask the dispenser for hearing aid insurance information. Some companies specifically underwrite policies for hearing aids.

8. *Hearing aid service.* Repairs and adjustments may be needed during the warranty period and for as long as you own the hearing aids. Also, your hearing may change, necessitating a change in the settings of your hearing aids. You want to be able to bring your hearing aids to the dispenser when you have a problem. Find out if you need to schedule an appointment or if you can walk in. If the hearing aids have to be sent to the manufacturer for repair, ask how long this usually takes and if you can use a loaner hearing aid during that time. Chapter 13 covers hearing aid repairs in more detail.

Being a Good Consumer

Choosing to buy hearing aids is an important decision. You want to have as much knowledge as possible to make an informed decision. Do not be afraid to ask the hearing aid dispenser questions. Most dispensers will give you a quote specifying the terms of purchase and you should read it before you sign anything. Do not be pressured by gimmicks such as a "one time only" sale or deal. A genuine sale price, or any price for that matter, should be guaranteed for a specified amount of time, not just for that moment.

Part of being a good consumer involves comparison shopping and being comfortable with a dispenser. You will be seeing a lot of that person and you want to feel you can trust him or her. Buying hearing aids is not like buying a television. You are buying that dispenser's expertise and services in addition to a product. Don't buy a mail-order hearing aid or a hearing aid out of someone's car trunk. You may find the same hearing aid costs several hundred dollars more from one dispenser to another. Take into account the experience, the reputation, the training, and the services offered when deciding where to purchase your hearing aids. You owe it to yourself to be a good, cautious consumer.

Chapter 9

Understanding Hearing Aids

Hearing aids have evolved from ear trumpets and large boxes with earphones that had to sit on a table to smaller and smaller wearable devices. Today's hearing aids easily fit behind or in the ear and the sound quality is better than at any other time in their history. Every few years brings another innovation in hearing aids, and these improvements will continue into the future. Hearing loss is one of the most common events of aging and there is at least a 30% chance that you will have a hearing loss and be able to benefit from a hearing aid if you are over 60 years of age. The more you know about hearing aids, the better prepared you are to purchase and use them effectively.

This chapter introduces you to hearing aids: what they do, how they work, the different styles and special features, and which hearing aids work best for different types of hearing losses. Current hearing aid technology, such as noise reduction circuitry and programmable hearing aids, also are covered. A summary of information for each hearing aid style is provided at the end of the chapter.

What Is a Hearing Aid?

A hearing aid is a small electronic device that picks up sound with a microphone, amplifies and filters it, and then conveys that sound into your ear canal through a loudspeaker, also called a receiver. The amplifiers in the hearing aid make sound louder. The filters selectively choose which pitches in the incoming sound will be emphasized. All of these components are miniaturized to fit inside a small case that is worn either behind or within your ear. Most hearing aids are custom molded to fit your ears from an impression taken by the dispenser. All hearing aids are powered by small batteries. Each hearing aid has a serial number registered by the manufacturer.

In general, hearing aids are either manufactured to match your hearing loss and/or they have controls the hearing aid dispenser adjusts to compensate for your loss. The features and controls your hearing aids have depend partly on what the manufacturer builds in and partly on what the dispenser orders for you. The appropriateness of the control settings depends a great deal on your dispenser's knowledge and expertise.

Hearing aids last an average of 5 years, although they can last longer with proper care and maintenance. Hearing aid technology changes and improves so you may want to replace them every 3 to 5 years.

What Do Hearing Aids Do and How Do They Work?

The primary purpose of hearing aids is to make sound louder. Since you have a hearing loss which makes sounds and speech too soft, you need a way to make them comfortably loud. Presbycusis usually causes some problem with speech clarity (discrimination) so ideally the hearing aids should make speech more clear, too. Both loudness and clarity are at least partially provided by hearing aids.

Hearing aids do not come in only one strength, adjustable for all hearing losses. The amount of amplification and the power of the hearing aid are different for different hearing losses. Therefore, the greater your hearing loss, the stronger the hearing aid. The volume control allows you to adjust the sound to a comfortable loudness within the total amount of power the hearing aid produces. All hearing aids limit the amount of amplification so that the very loud sounds they direct to your ears do not exceed a certain amount. In other words, a very loud noise will not be amplified proportionately as much as soft or normal sounds.

Hearing aids are constructed to amplify most of the pitches at which your hearing is tested. This is by design, of course, because you want the hearing aid to correct your hearing for the pitches at which speech sounds occur. Hearing aid filters are built to compensate for the range of pitches at which you have hearing loss, with the idea of improving your hearing equally for those pitches. This not only improves how you hear but also may improve your understanding (discrimination) of speech. Sometimes these filters are further adjustable by the dispenser for even greater control.

The theory of equalizing your hearing for all pitches with hearing aids makes sense, and it works well on paper. In reality, it is not that simple. Miniaturization of electronic parts and the complexity of the auditory (hearing) system and the brain limit the effectiveness of hearing aids in some situations and prevent this goal from being realized for every person and every hearing loss.

Why Do Hearing Aids Squeal?

This is worthy of special mention because everyone who knows anyone with a hearing aid has heard this rather unpleasant sound and wondered what it was. It is called feedback and it is a high-pitched squeal or whistle. Hearing aids emit this sound under certain conditions. Feedback is caused when amplified sound leaks back out of the ear canal and is reamplified by the hearing aid. It happens if the hearing aid is turned up too loud, if it is not fitting properly or if something (like a hat or a hand) is too close to the hearing aid. Feedback often alerts you to something that needs attention. More information on fixing feedback is found in Chapter 13.

Hearing Aids and Their Common Components

Hearing aids are available in several types or styles. The four most common styles will be discussed. All are shown in the illustrations that follow with their respective parts labeled. Styles numbered 1 through 3 below account for 98% of hearing aids sold today.

1. In-the-Ear (ITE)

2. In-the-Canal (ITC)

3. Behind-the-Ear (BTE)

4. Eyeglass

The components common to these hearing aid styles are covered in the next section. The common components are volume controls, user-operated switches, earmolds, and battery compartments.

Volume Controls

Volume controls usually are raised wheels with ridges that rotate in one direction to increase volume and in the opposite direction to decrease volume. You should be able to adjust the volume control of any hearing aid while it is in your ear. The volume controls on some BTE and eyeglass hearing aids have numbered positions to make setting them easier. The volume controls on in-the-ear (ITE) and in-the-canal (ITC) hearing aids are not numbered and usually click to the OFF position when the volume is turned all the way down. On BTE and eyeglass aids a separate switch usually turns the hearing aid to OFF. Volume control operation is covered in Chapter 11.

Some ITE and ITC aids have volume controls that are set by the dispenser and cannot be adjusted by the user. The drawback to this type of volume control is that you can't turn it louder or softer yourself.

User-Operated Switches

Switches are most commonly found on BTE and eyeglass hearing aids, although some ITEs have them too. Their purposes are to turn the hearing aid on and off, to turn on the telephone mode, and/or to turn on the noise reduction mode. Your fingertip slides the switch from one position to another.

ON-OFF and telephone switches are usually marked "O"-"M" or "O"-"T"-"M." The "O" position is always "OFF" and the "M" position activates the microphone and so turns the hearing aid on, or to the mode for listening to sound and speech. The "T" position activates the telecoil, which picks up and amplifies sound from the telephone. Instructions for using a hearing aid with the telephone are given in Chapter 11.

Some BTE and eyeglass aids have switches marked with letters such as "S," "L," "N," or "H." These designations refer to different frequency (pitch) amplification capabilities of the hearing aid and allow the user to select which he or she likes best in given situations. Different positions can be chosen when, for example, you are in a noisy place and would like to filter out more of the background sound. Then you would move the switch to the "S" or the "H" position, which decreases background, low pitched sound. In a quiet place you might choose the "L" or "N" position, which amplifies all pitches and makes speech sound more natural. The dispenser should familiarize you with each setting if you have hearing aids with these switches so that you know when to select each setting.

Earmolds

Earmolds are a component of BTE and eyeglass hearing aids which are custom-made to fit your ears. The dispenser takes an impression of each ear. Impression material is placed in each ear canal and is allowed to set up for 5 to 10 minutes. When the material is removed, it retains the shape of your ear. The dispenser sends the impressions to an earmold laboratory. The finished product is returned to the dispenser in a few days.

Earmolds are made of clear or tinted hard plastic (lucite) or of a variety of soft materials. Lucite earmolds may need to be replaced every few years if the plastic shrinks. Soft earmolds shrink more rapidly and may need replacement every year or two. Earmolds come in many shapes and styles based on your hearing loss. Earmolds may completely fill your ears or may be quite small and have an air channel, or vent, going through them. In general, the greater your hearing loss, the more the earmold will fill your ear. Milder and high frequency losses may be fitted with a smaller earmold. Earmolds on BTE and eyeglass aids have a clear plastic tubing which connects them to the hearing aids. This plastic tubing needs to be replaced once a year or when it becomes hard and yellowish.

Earmolds do more than simply anchor the hearing aids to your ears. Their shape, insertion depth into the ear canal, vent, and tubing all play an important part in the sound quality you hear through the hearing aids. Major adjustments of sounds are made through the hearing aids, but additional fine tuning of sound can be done with the earmolds.

Battery Compartments

All styles of hearing aids have battery compartments. Usually they swing out of the hearing aid case and the battery fits into the door. Battery compartments on some ITE and ITC aids are recessed into the hearing aid itself and close with a "toilet-seat" door. The battery is dropped into the compartment of these hearing aids.

All of these styles of hearing aids use small, round button-cell batteries. The battery size each style of hearing aid uses is summarized at the end of the chapter. Because batteries and their proper use are so important, they are covered in the next chapter, Understanding Hearing Aid Batteries.

Styles of Hearing Aids

Each hearing aid style is explained in the following sections. Information about the amount of hearing loss each corrects and special considerations for using them are also given.

In-the-Ear (ITE) Hearing Aids

ITE hearing aids (see illustration on the next page) are the most common type worn today. In-the-ear aids are so-called because they fill in the entire bowl portion of the outer ears (pinnae) and essentially plug into your ears. They must be custom molded, so the dispenser will take impressions of your ears. The manufacturer then builds the hearing aid cases, or shells, in the shape of the impressions so that the hearing aids fit the contours of your ears. In 1992, you could expect to pay from about $550 to $800 for one standard ITE aid.

Amount of Hearing Loss and ITE Aids

ITE hearing aids are appropriate for mild, moderate, and even moderate-to-severe hearing losses. They also have special applications for high-frequency hearing losses. Because of their relatively small size, they are somewhat

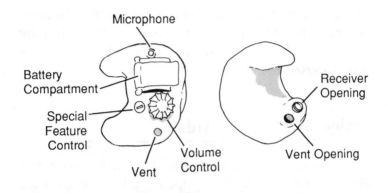

In-the-Ear (ITE) hearing aid. Left: Front view. Right: Back view.

limited in the amount of power and amplification they can produce. The more powerful ITEs are, the greater the possibility they will feed back in your ears.

The hearing aid dispenser should be honest with you about the severity of your hearing loss and using ITE aids. You should seriously consider BTE hearing aids if you have a severe hearing loss. If your hearing loss is profound, you should not use ITE aids at all. Manufacturers continue to develop stronger ITEs so that people with more severe hearing losses are able to use them, but feedback can still be a problem. Sometimes people with severe hearing losses who use ITEs have to keep them turned down so they don't squeal, but then they may not hear very well with them.

Other Considerations Before Purchasing ITEs

Some people are not able to use ITE hearing aids because of visual and physical dexterity limitations. Visual problems may prevent a person from seeing the hearing aid itself, the batteries, or the volume control. Physical limitations may prevent a person from being able to insert the aid into the ear and adjust the volume control.

If you are worried about these potential problems, try adjusting the volume control and inserting a battery on a model in your dispenser's office before you order one. Although a model will not fit in your ear since it is not made for you, you can try reaching it up to your ear to determine if you have enough finger dexterity and shoulder movement to do so.

In-the-Canal (ITC) Hearing Aids

ITC hearing aids (see illustration on page 106) are also custom molded and fit into the ear canal. They protrude slightly into the bowl of your outer ears but do not fill them. ITCs have been advertised as "invisible" hearing aids, though they are not. They became very popular in the 1980s after former President Reagan publicly proclaimed that he used one. ITCs are considered the most cosmetically appealing of hearing aids by consumers because of their small size, and every year ITC sales increase. Their small size, however, makes them more prone to repair problems, limits how powerful they can be, makes them harder to manipulate physically, and increases their cost. An ITC aid may cost up to twice as much as an ITE aid. The greater price is not because they are better quality, but because they are small and popular. In 1992, you could expect to pay $700 to $1500 for one ITC aid.

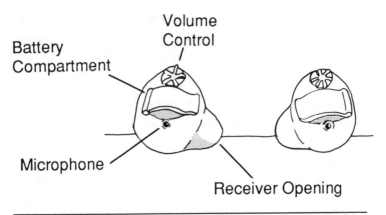

In-the-Canal (ITC) hearing aid: Front view.

Amount of Hearing Loss and ITC Aids

ITC hearing aids are appropriate for mild and moderate hearing losses, as well as for some high-frequency losses. Some moderate hearing losses may be borderline for using ITC hearing aids, and you might get better hearing loss correction for your money by using ITE or BTE aids. If you have a severe or profound hearing loss, ITC aids will not help you enough. Despite these drawbacks, people with severe or profound hearing losses have bought them on bad advice or from their desire to have small aids. More powerful ITCs are being developed, but, as with stronger ITE aids, stronger ITC hearing aids are more prone to feedback.

Miniaturization has limited the ability of ITC aids to fit all hearing losses, regardless of what some advertisements proclaim. They are too small to accommodate many amplifiers or filters. Yet, ITC aids do work for many people, and their small size makes people more motivated to use hearing aids when they would not otherwise do so.

Other Considerations Before Purchasing ITCs

The same considerations that apply to ITE aids also apply to ITC aids. Physical or visual limitations are even more important when considering ITC purchase, however. Good finger dexterity with little numbness in the fingertips is necessary to insert an ITC and turn the volume control. Taking an ITC aid out of the ear is more difficult than is taking out an ITE aid. If you have very large fingers, you may have trouble grasping and using an ITC aid and changing batteries. Again, try out these manipulations on a model in the dispenser's office to be sure you can do them before you order one.

Behind-the-Ear (BTE) Hearing Aids

Behind-the-ear hearing aids (see illustration on page 108) were the most popular hearing aid style in the 1960s and 1970s, but sales began to decline in the 1980s when ITE aids improved in performance and popularity. BTE hearing aids fit over and behind the ears, are anywhere from 1 to 2 inches in length, and couple to your ears with earmolds and small lengths of clear plastic tubing. They tuck easily behind most ears, even if you wear glasses. BTE case colors range from beige, brown, and grey to match hair color, all the way to green, yellow, orange, red, and blue for the more daring. BTE aids are usually fit on infants and children and still have wide applicability for adults. The larger size of BTE aids easily accommodates

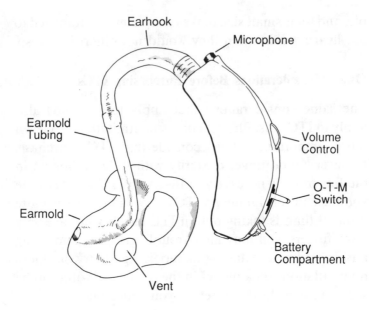

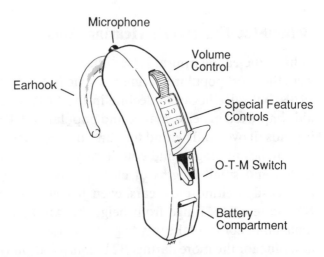

Behind-the-Ear (BTE) hearing aid with earmold. Top: Side view. Bottom: Back view.

amplifiers and filters which makes them more effective in the control of sound. BTE hearing aids generally need fewer repairs than ITE or ITC aids and may be more reliable. You could expect to pay $600 to $850 for one BTE aid in 1992.

Amount of Hearing Loss and BTE Aids

BTE hearing aids are the most versatile of all of the available styles because of the size and effectiveness of the electronic components and the earmold modification possibilities. BTEs accommodate all hearing losses from mild to profound and high-frequency losses. BTE aids designed for severe to profound hearing losses are very powerful, while BTE aids designed for milder losses are less powerful. BTE aids, especially powerful ones, may produce feedback but it is usually less of a problem than it is with other styles of hearing aids.

The hearing aid dispenser may tell you that you should have BTE aids for the best correction of your hearing loss. Certainly, if you have a severe-to-profound hearing loss, you should use BTE aids. Some high-frequency hearing losses may also be corrected better with BTE aids.

Other Considerations Before Purchasing BTEs

In general, the larger size of BTE hearing aids makes them easier to grasp with the fingers. The controls are larger than on ITE and ITC aids, so they are easier to see and feel. The larger battery used in some BTE aids is also easier to see and to hold between the fingers. However, because you have to deal with two pieces, the earmold and the BTE aid itself, it is easier for some people to insert a one-piece ITE aid. There really are not any hard and fast guidelines for which type is easier to handle physically, so try manipulating the parts of each style of hearing aid in the dispenser's office before making a decision.

Perhaps the greatest limitation of BTE aids is that you may reject them on the basis of their looks because you may feel they are more conspicuous than ITE aids. Their advantages, however, may outweigh cosmetic concerns in some cases, so try not to select hearing aids solely by their physical appearance.

Eyeglass Hearing Aids

Eyeglass hearing aids (see illustration on facing page) were very popular in the 1960s, but now represent a very small portion of the hearing aid market (fewer than 2% of sales). Manufacturers largely have dropped production of eyeglass aids, although some still make them. Part of their popularity was the perceived convenience of incorporating glasses with hearing aids. Also the style offered more concealment as BTE aids 30 years ago were larger than they are now and body-worn aids were still common. The waning of their popularity was due to improvements in BTE and ITE aids and to some problems unique to the eyeglass style. Eyeglass aids are built in the shape of the bows of glasses but are thicker and heavier than regular bows. They come in black, brown, and grey to match frame colors as closely as possible. Prices are similar to those of BTE aids.

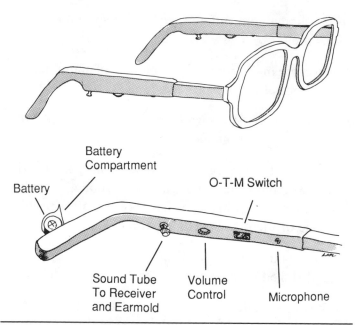

Battery
Compartment

Battery

O-T-M Switch

Sound Tube
To Receiver
and Earmold

Volume
Control

Microphone

Eyeglass hearing aid. Top: Full view. Bottom: Close-up view.

Amount of Hearing Loss and Eyeglass Aids

Eyeglass hearing aids are appropriate for mild through severe hearing losses and for high-frequency losses, just as BTE aids are. It is still possible to order eyeglass aids that fit all of these hearing losses, but the special features available are limited, because so few are being produced.

Other Considerations Before Purchasing Eyeglass Aids

The eyeglass style hearing aid presents some special considerations not applicable to other styles. Even so, some people are satisfied with eyeglass hearing aids and prefer not to change to a different style. The special consider-ations are:

1. Fewer are made now so fewer choices of manufacturers and special features are available.

2. They should be considered only if you wear your glasses all the time, not just for reading.

3. Your glasses cannot be separated from your hearing aids with this style, so you can't wear your glasses alone or your hearing aids alone. This is especially a problem if one or the other needs repair.

4. They make your glasses heavy and they press down on the bridge of your nose harder than regular glasses.

5. They limit your choice of glasses frames because they are relatively thick and only come in three colors.

6. Your glasses will probably need to be modified so the hearing aid adaptors will fit properly when connected to the frames. This could require trips to both the dis-penser and the optician. Not all hearing aid dispensers are comfortable with or skilled in modifying glasses. And, not all opticians are comfortable modifying glasses with hearing aids in them.

7. Even with proper modifications, your glasses may not fit as snugly against your head because they can't be bent as much as regular bows.

8. With all of the above considerations, some hearing aid dispensers do not even sell eyeglass hearing aids.

Variations of ITE, BTE, and Eyeglass Hearing Aids: CROS Style Aids

CROS is an acronym for Contralateral Routing of Sound. These hearing aids were developed for people with a severe to profound hearing loss in one ear and normal or near-normal hearing in the better ear. They look like two hearing aids but are actually one split into two parts. The principle of a CROS hearing aid is to put the microphone on the poorer ear to pick up sound on that side of the head and transmit it to the other ear so that the sound is heard in the better ear for optimal sound interpretation. Wearing a CROS style aid may also restore your ability to localize sound direction. The transmission of sound from one side of the head to the other is accomplished either by a wire or by radio signal. Both sides of the hearing aid must be worn because they function together as a single unit. This is useful when, for example, there is no hearing in your poor ear and it would not help to put a hearing aid on that ear, but you would still like to hear sound from that side.

If your better ear has some hearing loss and you need amplification, you can wear a BI-CROS aid, which provides amplification for the better ear. If you have normal or near-normal hearing in your better ear, you can wear a CROS aid, which only gives minimal amplification in the better ear.

Special Options Available in Hearing Aids

Hearing aids can have special options, or features, built into them. These options control the sounds you hear through the hearing aid, primarily by additional filtering and loudness moderation. This section describes the special options that are currently available. Not all are appropriate for all hearing losses and not all are available for each style of hearing aid. In general, the larger the hearing aid, the greater the number of special options it can accommodate. Therefore, BTE hearing aids may have more features than ITE aids, and ITC aids can accommodate very few. Eyeglass hearing aids have fewer special options than BTE aids since so few are being manufactured. You should discuss the options available with your dispenser when you order your hearing aids and decide which would be most helpful for your particular hearing loss. These options usually add to the cost of the hearing aid.

1. *Tone Control.* A tone control is a filter that adjusts the amount of low-frequency (pitch) amplification the hearing aid produces. Some hearing aids also have a similar control for high-frequency amplification. This allows the dispenser to adjust the hearing aid to either amplify a broad range of pitches or a more specific range of pitches, based on your hearing loss and your listening preference.

2. *Feedback Control.* The function of a feedback control is to reduce the feedback squeal, which can be a problem in strong hearing aids and in very high-frequency emphasis hearing aids.

3. *Power Control.* This control should not be confused with the volume control that all hearing aids have and that the user adjusts. The power control is set by the dispenser to vary the amount of power and amplification the hearing aid produces so that it does not have to always be

at full strength. Operating a hearing aid at full strength also uses batteries faster. The hearing aids selected for you may have more power than you need, so that if your hearing should get worse the power can be increased and you won't need to buy new, stronger hearing aids right away.

4. *Compression Circuits.* Automatic Gain Control (AGC), Input and Output Compression, and Frequency Dependent Compression are some of the options available. Compression circuits decrease the volume, or gain, a hearing aid produces as the surrounding level of sound increases. Compression circuits turn themselves on and off, depending on the level and pitch of the noise you are in. These types of controls function to reduce overall amplification of noise and speech in noisy environments.

5. *Adaptive Circuits for Noise Reduction or Speech Enhancement.* Automatic Signal or Speech Processing (ASP), K-Amp™, Noise Blockers, and Noise Suppression Controls are examples. These circuits continue to be improved and a great deal of research time and money are spent on them. The purpose of all of these circuits is to reduce background noise interference, primarily by reducing low-frequency (pitch) amplification, thus making speech easier to hear and understand. The K-Amp™ works differently and primarily amplifies soft, high-frequency sounds without amplifying loud sounds. Adaptive circuits work automatically although, in some cases, you may have a switch to turn them on when you are in a noisy place.

Adaptive circuits can be quite effective in reducing the sharpness of background noise and in filtering some of it out. They do not filter or block out all background noise, however. It is still not possible to eliminate all background noise without also filtering out too many speech sounds. In some cases, these circuits have been marketed erroneously as eliminating background noise. Consumers may purchase them with the expectation that they won't hear background noise but will hear and understand words clearly, and are disappointed. If you know what the circuits can and can't do, your expectations of their performance will be more realistic. Even though these circuits do not eliminate all background noise, they make listening through hearing aids manageable and pleasant for many people. Ask your dispenser which of them would be most appropriate for you.

6. *Push-Pull Circuitry and Dual Receivers.* Both of these options increase the power hearing aids can produce while keeping the sound clear. For example, when you turn up your TV volume too high, it gets loud but the sound is distorted and not clear. The same can happen with hearing aids. These engineering developments allow greater power with a high fidelity sound quality.

7. *Telecoil (T-Coil).* The T-coil option enables you to use a telephone more effectively or to connect your hearing aid to a special listening system found in some churches and public buildings. The T-coil is usually standard on BTE and eyeglass hearing aids. A T-coil can be added to ITE aids, space permitting, but is not available on ITC aids. The T-coil amplifies the magnetic field around a telephone, so that you hear the person's voice more loudly and clearly. Some telephones have no magnetic leakage,

however, so check with your phone company for T-coil compatibility before purchasing this option.

8. *Direct Audio Input.* Direct audio input enables you to plug your hearing aids into listening systems, TVs, radios, or other audio equipment. This direct connection amplifies the sound you are listening to more precisely and decreases or eliminates competing background noise. This option is usually available only in BTE aids.

9. *Digital and Programmable Circuits.* These relatively new concepts in hearing aid circuitry are available in BTE ITE and ITC aids from several manufacturers. Hearing aids with these circuits are programmed either by computer or other specialized equipment in the dispenser's office. They may offer more exact correction of your hearing loss than traditional hearing aids by more precisely amplifying the pitches at which you have hearing loss. Their noise control ability may also be superior. Most of the currently available hearing aids with programmable and digital circuits have several settings which the dispenser programs. A remote control panel allows selection of the settings. You may have one setting you prefer for quiet places, one for noisy places, one for listening to music, and so on. These may be the "wave of the future" and you probably can expect them to become more common. Hearing aids with digital and programmable circuits cost substantially more than traditional hearing aids. You may expect to pay from $1,500 to $2,500 per hearing aid in 1992.

Because so much has been presented in this chapter and because hearing aids are such a complex topic, a sum-

Summary of Hearing Aid Styles and Indications for Use

Style	Cost in 1992	Battery Size/Life	Special Features Available	Hearing Loss
ITE	$550-$800	13 or 312 1-4 weeks	1, 2, 3, 4, 5 6, 7, 9	Mild, Moderate, or Severe
ITC	$700-$1,500	312 or 10 3 days- 4 weeks	1, 2, 3, 4, 5 9	Mild, Moderate, or Moderate-to-Severe
BTE	$600-$850	13 or 675 3 days- 4 weeks	1, 2, 3, 4, 5 6, 7, 8, 9	Mild, Moderate, Severe, or Profound
Eyeglass	$700-$850	13 or 675 3 days- 4 weeks	1, 3, 4, 7	Mild, Moderate, or Severe

mary is provided to review the different styles of hearing aids and their characteristics. The special feature numbers listed refer to those explained in this section, with the corresponding description number.

Hearing aids are small packages that enable you to hear people talking and to hear the sounds in your environment again. Hearing aid research to reproduce the sounds

you do want to hear more exactly and to reduce the
sounds you don't want to hear continues. We can all look
forward to more hearing aid innovations as time goes on.

Chapter 10

Understanding Hearing Aid Batteries

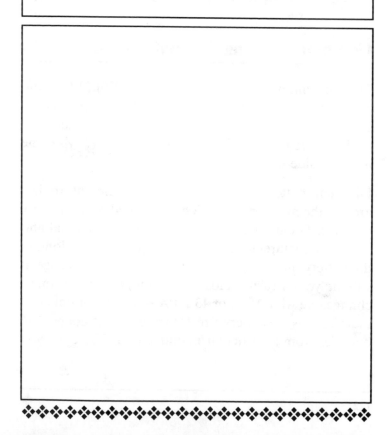

All hearing aids require a power source which is provided by small, round, button-cell batteries. Batteries are an integral part of your hearing aids and understanding them is necessary for optimal hearing aid performance.

This chapter discusses the common button-cell battery sizes, the materials they are made from, their expected life span, where they can be purchased, their care, battery safety, and tips for prolonging their use. Rechargeable built-in batteries, used by a few manufacturers, are not discussed as they are uncommon. Rechargeable batteries are uncommon because they frequently malfunction, are difficult to service, and expensive to replace.

Common Hearing Aid Battery Sizes

The four common battery sizes are 10 (or 230), 312, 13, and 675. The actual sizes are shown in the illustration on page 123. Each battery has a negative and positive side. The positive side is flat and is stamped with a "+" while the negative side has a raised circle.

Different battery manufacturers use different initials around the number size which is stamped on the battery package. The initials designate the battery material and that manufacturer's particular coding system. As long as the battery number you need appears on the package, it will fit your hearing aids. For example, 13A is interchangeable with AC13 or 13 HPX — it is the number 13 that signifies the battery size. Hearing aids do not require batteries from a particular manufacturer. Therefore you

ACTUAL BATTERY SIZE

	10 or 230	312	13	675
Negative Side	▭	▭	▭	▭
Positive Side	⊕	+	+	+
	For ITC Hearing Aids	For ITC, ITE and some BTE Hearing Aids	For ITE, BTE and Eyeglass Hearing Aids	For BTE and Eyeglass Hearing Aids

Common hearing aid batteries

can use Duracell and Eveready and Ray-O-Vac, and other brands, interchangeably.

The number size is critical regardless of where you buy the batteries or which company manufactures them. If you buy the wrong sized batteries, your hearing aids will not work. Be especially careful with sizes 13 and 312, which look similar. If your hearing aids take a size 13 battery, you may not substitute a size 312.

Battery Materials

Hearing aid batteries are most commonly made of either zinc or mercury. It does not matter which type you use (as long as the battery is the correct size). Each material has different performance characteristics, however.

1. *Mercury (Mercuric-Oxide) Batteries.* These batteries provide reliable service and are the least expensive. They last only about half as long as zinc-air batteries in the same hearing aid. Hearing aid manufacturers feel that they may provide more reliable performance for very strong hearing aids and for any hearing aid in humid weather. These batteries have a relatively short shelf life (about one year) so you should purchase them from a store that sells a lot of batteries or restocks them frequently to reduce the chance of buying a bad pack. They usually come in a package of six, and there are regular and premium options. The premium mercury batteries last longer than the regular ones.

As of 1991, Vermont and Minnesota had banned batteries containing mercury as a potential environmental hazard. At least four other states are considering banning them. Mercury batteries could become more difficult to find if battery legislation becomes more common.

2. *Zinc-Air Batteries.* These batteries come with an adhesive tab on them to cover tiny air holes. Once the tab is removed, the battery is activated and ready for use. You should discard the tab since putting it back on does not deactivate the battery. You should *not* remove the battery tab until you are ready to use a new one. Zinc-air batteries

have more material packed into them and they last twice as long as mercury batteries in the same hearing aid. Each zinc-air battery is more expensive than a mercury battery, but the cost is not twice as much. This makes zinc-air batteries more cost effective to use. Zinc-air batteries come in packages of three, four, or six and have regular and premium options. They also have a longer shelf life (about 5 years) than mercury batteries, so you are less likely to buy a bad pack.

Battery Life

A hearing aid battery may last from a few days to four weeks. Major manufacturers are introducing "low-drain" circuits in some of their models, which can double battery life, but they are not yet commonly available. The relatively short life span of a hearing aid battery is usually surprising to most new hearing aid users. Hearing aids require substantially more power to perform the functions of amplifying and filtering sound than do a watch or a calculator to perform their functions. It is true that batteries are an ongoing expense, but you should not let that deter you from using your hearing aids and reaping the benefits they provide. After all, you don't let your car sit in the garage because driving it uses gas.

The battery life of your hearing aids depends on the circuit drain (the current needed to power the circuits), how strong your hearing aids are, the hours of use per day, the material the battery is made from (zinc-air lasts about twice as long as mercury), and the size of the battery. A stronger hearing aid uses batteries faster than a milder strength hearing aid. And, in general, the larger the battery size, the longer the battery lasts. Your dispenser should provide you with the battery life you can expect when you get your hearing aids.

Hearing aid batteries "die" a couple of different ways. The hearing aid may get weaker and weaker, requiring you to keep increasing the volume. This is more typical of a mercury battery. Or batteries will keep their full power and die suddenly, often making a distorted, motor-boating sound on their way out. This is more typical of a zinc-air battery. You know your battery is dead or dying when:

1. No amplification is present.

2. The hearing aid no longer squeals when you hold it cupped in your hand.

3. The sound is weaker and you have to keep turning the aid up louder.

4. You hear a motor-boating or static sound.

Purchasing Hearing Aid Batteries

Hearing aid batteries are easy to find. Batteries are available from your hearing aid dispenser and many dispensers mail them upon request or have battery club booklets. They can be purchased from pharmacies and discount stores and are even available from some grocery stores. You can also find them in electronics stores (such as Radio Shack). Some senior citizens organizations offer battery specials too. A package of batteries may cost anywhere from $4.00 to $12.00 depending on the material they are made from and where you purchase them. It's a good idea to price shop for batteries since you'll be buying them regularly over the years.

Battery Care, Storage, and Disposal

Batteries should be stored at room temperature, in a safe, dry place. Do not store them near heat and do not store them in the refrigerator or freezer. If you keep them cold, moisture will condense on them and that can introduce moisture into the hearing aid.

Dispose of batteries properly in your trash or, better yet, recycle them. Battery recycling programs exist but they are not common. If your dispenser does not know of a battery recycling program, call your local recycling center and inquire. Most hearing aid batteries are disposed of in landfills and that is why mercury batteries are being outlawed in some states. Supposedly, zinc-air batteries are environmentally benign when disposed of.

Battery Safety and
The National Battery Hotline

Batteries contain chemicals, and they should be treated with proper respect. Five safety issues should be considered.

1. Batteries are very harmful to your health (and that of infants and pets) if they are swallowed. If a battery has been swallowed, call a doctor immediately and pro-ceed to an Emergency Room. For recommended treat-

ment, contact the National Battery Hotline (collect) at (202)-625-3333.

2. Store and discard batteries in places where infants, small children, and pets cannot get to them.

3. Do not store batteries where they may be mistaken for pills.

4. Do not dispose of batteries in incinerators or fires because they can rupture and explode.

5. If batteries show any sign of leakage, dispose of them immediately.

Leakage may appear as a white material around the raised, negative side. Battery corrosion usually is green and corroded batteries should also be discarded. Old batteries are the most likely to have leakage. If batteries are even a year old, you should inspect them before putting them into your hearing aids.

Battery Tips

The following tips will help you get the best possible battery life and use:

1. Open the battery compartment of your hearing aid whenever it is not in use. Some hearing aids drain battery power even when they are turned off (like flashlights) and battery life can be increased by disconnecting it. Opening the battery compartment also allows moisture to evaporate from the hearing aid.

2. Always carry spare batteries with you.

3. Do not carry loose batteries in your pocket or purse where they may contact metal objects such as coins, keys, or other batteries. This can cause them to discharge and die.

4. Keep the tabs on zinc-air batteries until you are ready to use one and only use one battery at a time.

5. Use new, fresh batteries for best hearing aid performance. Old batteries do not last long in your hearing aid and may leak chemicals.

6. Dispose of your dead batteries immediately so you don't confuse them with your new ones.

7. Insert batteries into the battery door carefully and do not force them in. Line up the "+" sign of the battery with the "+" sign on the battery door. See Chapter 11 for further information about correct battery insertion.

Chapter 11

Obtaining and Maintaining Your Hearing Aids

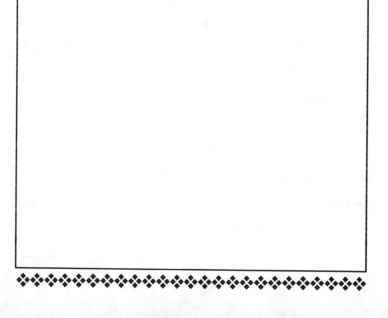

Hearing aid dispensers use the term "Hearing Aid Fitting" to describe picking up your new hearing aids, physically fitting them in your ears, and teaching you how to use them and care for them. This chapter takes you through these steps. Follow-up visits with the dispenser are also discussed. The information prepares you if you are planning on getting hearing aids and is a good review if you already have them. Caregivers and family members should read this chapter in order to help the hearing aid user at home.

Learning About Your Hearing Aids

When you get your new hearing aids, the dispenser will acquaint you with their parts and their use. If you think you will have physical difficulty handling the hearing aids or if you think you may forget important information, take someone along with you. It's important to have the support of friends and family, so if you need help once you get home, you can work on it with that person. Taking a support person with you also gives that person the chance to learn more about hearing aids and communication.

Your dispenser will teach you how to:

1. Insert and remove the hearing aids.

2. Turn them on and off.

3. Adjust the volume controls.

4. Use the telephone with your hearing aids.

5. Change batteries.

6. Clean and care for the hearing aids.

Since you and the dispenser will work on one hearing aid at a time, the fitting procedures will be discussed as if you only have one aid. The instructions also apply if you have two hearing aids.

Physical Fitting of the Hearing Aid

The hearing aid dispenser will first put the hearing aid in your ear to check the physical fit. The hearing aid or ear-mold was made in the shape of the ear impression that was taken when you ordered the aid. Occasionally some imperfections in the process occur and the fit may not be exact.

The hearing aid or earmold should:

1. Feel and look secure and snug in your ear.

2. Feel like you have something in your ear.

3. Not be uncomfortably tight.

4. Not be so loose that it dislodges or falls out when you move your head.

5. Not be painful or have rough or sharp edges.

The dispenser can assess the physical fit by looking at the hearing aid in your ear, but you are the only one who can tell if it is truly comfortable. Sometimes it has to be worn a few hours or days to fully determine how comfortable it is.

If any soreness, red spots, or open sores develop in your ear, contact your dispenser immediately and stop wearing the hearing aid. These can occur if there is some imperfection in the hearing aid or earmold. The dispenser can grind and buff it for a more comfortable fit. In some cases the aid or earmold may even need to be remade.

In time, you should barely be aware of the hearing aid in your ear, but at first you will be very conscious of it and you may even feel as if your ear is plugged up. The more you wear your hearing aid, the sooner you will get used to how it feels in your ear.

Insertion and Removal of the Hearing Aid

It is difficult to explain how to insert and remove a hearing aid because you need to experience it physically. It is desirable to be able to do these manuevers by feel but you may also find a mirror is helpful. Properly inserted ITE and ITC hearing aids are shown in the illustrations on page 135 and 136, and a properly inserted earmold with a BTE aid is shown in the illustration on page 137 (an earmold with an eyeglass aid is inserted the same way). Regardless of whether you have an ITE or an ITC hearing aid or a hearing aid with an earmold, the steps are the same. With practice, you will develop your own style. These suggestions are offered as a general guideline.

To insert the hearing aid:

1. Be sure the hearing aid is turned off to prevent feedback during insertion.

2. Orient the hearing aid or earmold so that the long portion with the hole(s) is at the bottom as you hold it. Refer to the illustration on page 138 for proper orienta-

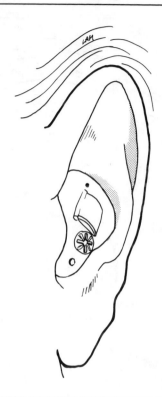

Proper Position of an In-the-Ear (ITE) hearing aid.

tion. If you have a BTE, let the hearing aid dangle
freely and just grasp the earmold with your fingers. If
you have an eyeglass aid, put the glasses on first, then
insert the earmold.

3. Bring the aid or earmold up to your ear without twisting
   your wrist. It helps to guide it along your cheek until
   you reach your ear.
4. Insert the long portion with the hole(s) into your ear
   canal. You should feel the aid or earmold sliding down

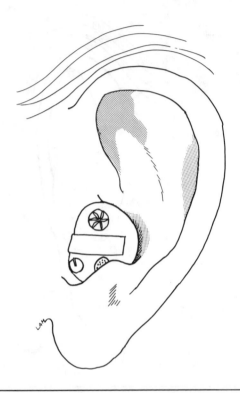

Proper position of an In-the-Canal (ITC) hearing aid.

into your ear. Use your other hand to pull up and back on your outer ear to open up your ear canal for easier insertion.

5. Twist the aid or earmold toward the back of your head while pushing it gently into your ear until it is in place. It may almost pop into the proper position.

6. If you have a BTE aid, then tuck the hearing aid over and behind your ear, as if you were tucking back a piece of hair.

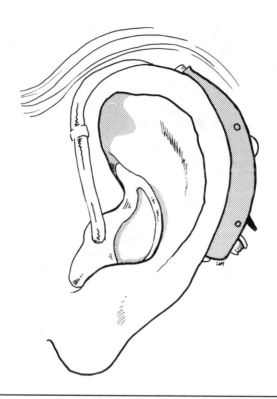

Proper position of a Behind-the-Ear (BTE) hearing aid.

7. Check in the mirror or by feeling to make sure that the aid is properly positioned (refer to the illustrations on pages 135, 136 and 137) and that no portion of the aid or earmold is sticking out of your ear. Your hearing aid will not fall out if it is inserted properly.

To remove the hearing aid:

1. Turn off the hearing aid to prevent feedback during removal.

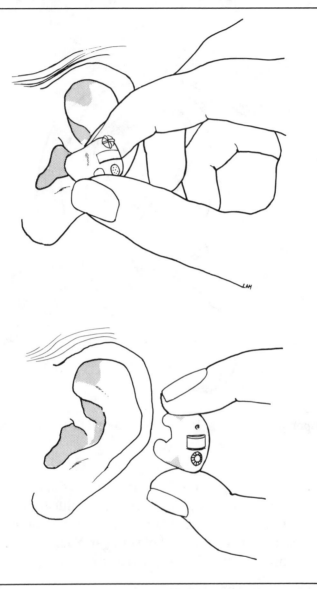

Proper orientation for hearing aid insertion.

2. Try to hook your thumb under the hearing aid or ear-mold and gently pry it out a bit.

3. Grasp it and pull it out of your ear.

4. If you have an earmold, you can pull gently where the tubing inserts into the earmold until it comes out of your ear. However, this causes the tubing to wear out faster and sometimes to become unglued. Steps 2 and 3 are better methods.

Turning the Hearing Aid On and Off

These functions can be performed while the hearing aid is in your ear. If there is an ON-OFF switch, such as on a BTE or eyeglass aid, practice sliding it on and off so you can do it quickly and easily. If the ON-OFF positions are built into the volume controls, such as with ITE and ITC aids, put your fingertip on the volume control and rotate it while maintaining a slight pressure for traction. The illustration on page 141 demonstrates this manuever. You may hear or feel it click on and off. Again, practice this action until you can do it easily and quickly.

Adjusting the Volume Control

An early goal should be learning to adjust the volume control while the hearing aid is in your ear. It takes some practice but is worth the effort because you will want to reach the most comfortable volume quickly depending on the situation you are in. Volume controls rotate differently, but most commonly:

1. Rotate the volume control clockwise to increase volume and counter-clockwise to decrease volume on an ITE or ITC hearing aid (see illustration on the facing page).

2. Rotate the volume control toward the top of the instrument to increase volume and down to decrease volume on most BTE aids. BTE aids also may have numbered positions with the smallest number being the softest and the largest number being the loudest.

3. Rotate the volume control toward the front of your glasses to decrease volume and toward the back of your glasses to increase volume on an eyeglass aid.

Try not to get caught up in thinking about clockwise versus counter-clockwise, up versus down, or front versus back. Concentrate on listening to whether the hearing aid is getting louder or softer rather than memorizing which way to rotate the volume control.

Where to Set the Volume Control

The dispenser may give you a specific volume setting based on tests done in the office. However, once you are wearing your hearing aid in the "real world" you may find that the setting needs to be changed. Some general guidelines exist for setting sound at a comfortable loudness. Comfortably loud sound means you can tell things sound louder than they normally do and you can hear sounds and voices more easily, but not so loudly that you jump

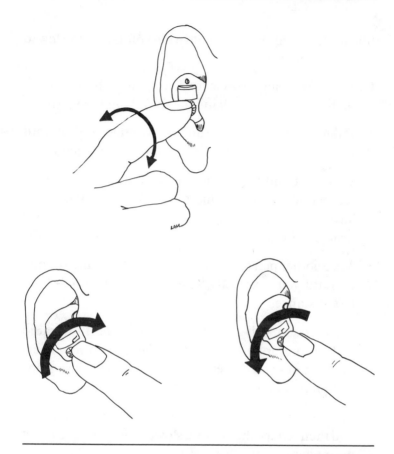

Top: Adjusting the volume control on an In-the-Ear (ITE) hearing aid. Bottom: Turning the hearing aid on and off.

or wince in response to them. Also, your own voice should sound louder to you (your voice is closest to the hearing aid after all) but not so loud that it echoes in your head. On the other hand, if your surroundings sound "normal," turn the volume up. "Normal" to you is a hearing loss and may mean you have the volume set too low to improve your hearing.

Here are some suggestions for setting the volume control if you have difficulty judging the sounds you are hearing.

1. Talk out loud while rotating the volume control until your own voice sounds louder, but doesn't echo.

2. Select a sound in your home (such as a clock chime, refrigerator or furnace motor, or TV or radio) that you have difficulty hearing and turn the volume of your hearing aid up until you can hear that sound easily.

3. Ask another person to talk to you and turn the volume up until you can easily hear that person at a 3- to 6-foot distance.

4. Ask a person with good hearing to turn the TV or radio on to a comfortable loudness. Then turn up your hearing aid until you can easily hear it too. This also stops complaints that you turn the TV up too loud.

5. Increase the volume of the hearing aid until it squeals, and then reduce the volume slowly until the squeal just disappears.

6. Hearing aid manufacturers suggest that you turn the volume to about one-half of full-on.

If you have two hearing aids, you ideally want to hear the same from each. Use these guidelines, but adjust both hearing aids so that the sounds you are listening to seem as if they are directly in front of you rather than sounding as if they are coming into just one ear. If you have numbered volume controls, try setting them at the same number. You can use a sound, such as rubbing your fingertips together next to each aid, to judge whether or not the sound is equally loud in each ear. Usually you don't need to turn two hearing aids up as loud to hear well as you do if you have only one hearing aid.

Naturally, the volume you find comfortable in one situation may not be appropriate for another. You may turn up the volume of your hearing aid in quiet situations and turn it down in loud situations. It is necessary to adjust the volume for comfort for the environment you are in. However, try to find a comfortable setting and leave it there until you change environments. Try not to constantly adjust the volume control.

Using the Telephone with Your Hearing Aid

Two ways of using the telephone with a hearing aid are described in detail: using the microphone of the hearing aid and using the "T" switch if your aid has one.

Using the Microphone with the Telephone

The microphone of the hearing aid is what picks up the sounds you listen to, so that means you must hold the telephone receiver near the microphone of the hearing aid. If you have a BTE aid, hold the telephone receiver above your ear, at the microphone opening. Hold the phone receiver at the microphone opening on the bow if you have an eyeglass aid. In some cases, you may be able to hold the phone at your earmold, but the earmold often blocks the person's voice from being heard.

When you hold the telephone to the microphone of an ITC or ITE aid, it may cause the hearing aid to feed back, or squeal. If that happens, hold the receiver away from your ear until the squeal disappears. The illustration below shows the way to hold the telephone with an ITC and an ITE hearing aid. Your dispenser may sell small foam pads that stick to the telephone receiver and provide extra space between it and the hearing aid, thus preventing feedback.

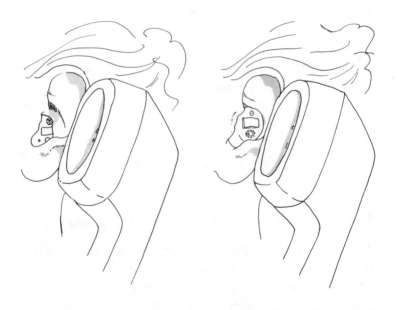

Using the telephone. Left: With an In-the-Canal (ITC) hearing aid. Right: With an In-the-Ear (ITE) hearing aid.

Using the Telecoil or
"T" Switch with the Telephone

Most BTE and eyeglass hearing aids come with a telecoil and the switch is labeled "T." If you ordered the telephone option on your ITE hearing aid, the control will be a small sliding switch on the front of the aid. When you move the switch to the telephone mode, the microphone is turned off and you no longer hear the sounds in your environment coming through the hearing aid. Instead a coil inside the hearing aid is activated which amplifies only the voice on the telephone. It is often helpful to turn up the volume control on the hearing aid when you use the telephone switch. Not all telephones are compatible with hearing aid telecoils. Those that are compatible are labeled.

If you have an ITE hearing aid, simply put the telephone up to your ear to listen. You must hold the telephone near the location of the telecoil in a BTE or eyeglass aid. The coil is usually located toward the bottom of the hearing aid of the BTE or at the back of the bow in an eyeglass aid. The illustration on page 146 shows the proper position of the telephone receiver when using the "T" switch on a BTE hearing aid.

Using the telephone with your hearing aid takes practice, regardless of whether you use a "T" switch or the microphone. It helps to practice with a friend who will call you and let you take the time to find the proper position of the phone with the hearing aid. You may also call a prerecorded message, such as the weather report, for practice.

Some people prefer to use an amplifier telephone that has a volume control built into the receiver rather than their

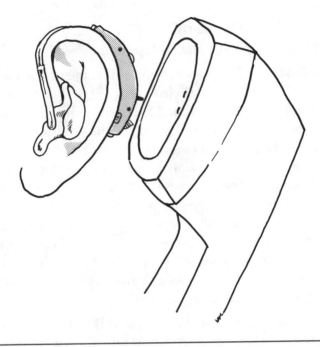

Using the telephone with a Behind-the-Ear (BTE) hearing aid set on the "T" switch position.

hearing aid. An amplifier telephone can be purchased from your telephone company, a telephone store, or from companies that sell products for people with hearing loss (see Chapter 14).

Changing the Batteries

Your dispenser will show you the battery door and have you practice inserting and removing the battery. The illus-

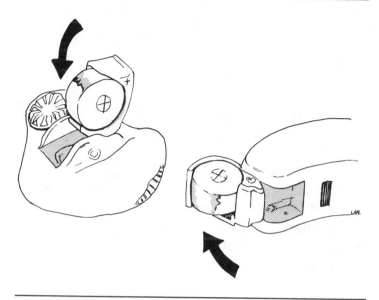

Correct battery insertion.

tration above shows batteries inserted into the doors of an ITE and a BTE hearing aid. You should make sure that you know the correct battery size. A battery fits only one way into the hearing aid, and the hearing aid will not work if the battery is not inserted correctly. If you invert it, the battery door may not close; and if you force it closed, the battery may be jammed inside the compartment. Most battery doors are marked with a "+" indicating that the positive side of the battery (also marked with a "+") should face that direction.

Your dispenser should give you information about how long you can expect a battery to last in your hearing aid. This is helpful to know so that you can anticipate when you will need a new battery. You should, with practice, recognize when your battery is dead or dying (see Chapter 10).

Care and Maintenance of Your Hearing Aid

Proper care and maintenance of your hearing aid prolongs its life and ensures that you get the best sound quality. Care and maintenance also minimize your trips into the dispenser's office. However, if you have physical or visual problems that prevent you from cleaning it or if you have no support person to help you at home, you should bring the hearing aid to the dispenser for regular cleaning. It is also possible to clean a hearing aid too vigorously and damage it. In this case, the dispenser may prefer you to bring the aid in for cleaning.

The following are some guidelines for care and maintenance of your hearing aid:

1. *Every day* you should wipe your hearing aid or earmold off with a soft cloth or tissue to keep skin oils, wax, and dirt from building up.

2. Use a wax loop and/or a brush (see illustration on the next page) to clean the holes in the hearing aid or earmold and pick out any wax accumulating in them. This should be done whenever you notice any debris in the holes of the hearing aid or earmold. This may be daily or occasionally, depending on how much wax your ears produce. If you can't get the wax out of the aid and the hearing aid is plugged up, have your dispenser clean it. Try not to jam

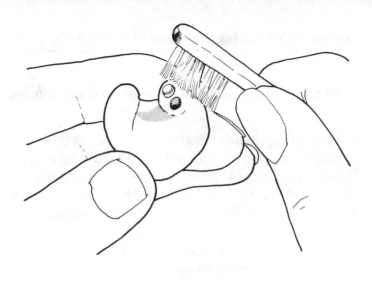

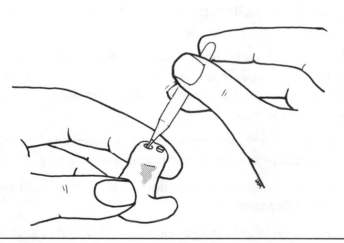

Cleaning a hearing aid. Top: With a brush. Bottom: With a wax loop.

the wax deeper into the holes because this could damage the aid.

If your hearing aid has an earmold (BTE or eyeglass aid), you can disconnect the earmold from the hearing aid (see illustration on page 151) for cleaning. Do this if you are unable to clean it effectively with a brush or wax loop. Wash the earmold (*not* the hearing aid) in warm, soapy water and use a pipe cleaner to swivel around in the hole(s) to get debris out. Rinse, shake out the excess water, and allow the earmold to dry overnight. Earmolds can also be soaked in denture cleaner to deodorize them.

3. Always open the battery door when your aid is not in use.

4. Store your hearing aid in a safe, room-temperature, dry place. A bureau drawer or a container are good storage places.

5. Store your batteries in a safe, dry place too. Go to an Emergency Room if you or someone else swallows a battery. Chapter 10 has specific information about battery safety and storage.

6. Schedule a yearly appointment to have your hearing aid checked for proper functioning and cleaning.

There are some important "don'ts" in hearing aid care and maintenance too.

1. *Do not get your hearing aid wet!* Never wash it or soak it in any solutions. Do not wipe it off with alcohol or disinfectant unless you have been directed to do so for health reasons. Do not wear it in the shower or when swimming and remember to take it off if you get your hair done.

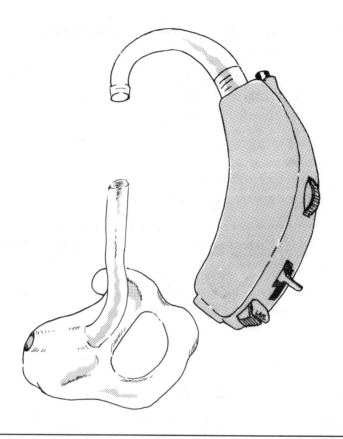

The earmold can be disconnected from the hearing aid for cleaning.

2. Do not store your hearing aid in the bathroom where steam from the shower can permeate it.

3. Do not use your hearing aid when you are sweating a lot, such as during exercise, heavy manual work, or even gardening if you are hot. Sweat evaporates into and even

flows into the hearing aid. Sweat is more corrosive than water because of the salts in it.

4. Do not drop your hearing aid or jar it on hard surfaces as it can break open or the circuitry inside can become disconnected.

5. Do not spray hairspray on the hearing aid. Take your aid off before spraying your hair and let the spray settle and dry before putting it back on. Hair spray can gum up the volume control, switches, and the microphone.

6. Do not store your hearing aid where heat can damage it, such as in direct sunlight, in the glove compartment of a car, or under a lamp.

7. Do not leave your hearing aid where small children or pets can get it. Pets eat hearing aids and children may swallow batteries.

Follow-up Visits with Your Dispenser

Follow-up visits with your dispenser are important for both you and the dispenser. You need to report your hearing experiences, both successful and unsuccessful, to your dispenser. He or she may be able to offer suggestions to solve problems and will enjoy sharing in your successes. If readjustments need to be made, the follow-up visits are the time to make them.

Your hearing aid dispenser should be available for questions or problems, or even for practicing insertion of the aid or adjusting the volume control. Your dispenser wants you to be as pleased as possible with your hearing aids and wants to make your listening experience enjoyable. If something isn't right, you must let the dispenser know. Don't feel that you are bothering the dispenser with questions — that is part of his or her job. A problem can't be remedied if it's not reported.

Chapter 12

Adjusting to
Your Hearing Aids

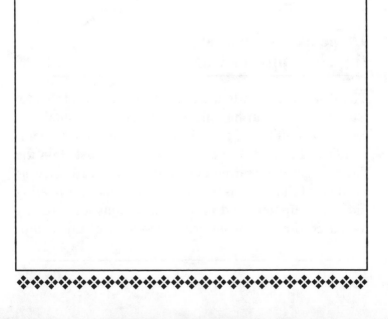

Hearing aids open up a whole new world of sounds. You hear things you didn't even realize you were missing. You hear sounds and voices, including your own, differently. Adjusting to the hearing aids and to a different way of hearing is an experience unique to each person. Every person adapts at different rates, some within a few days and others within a year or longer. And, unfortunately, some people never adjust to them or accept them. The way the hearing aids sound to you and proper adjustment of the controls to provide the best correction of your hearing loss are crucial in your acceptance of the hearing aids.

This chapter explains how the dispenser adjusts your hearing aids and verifies correction of your hearing loss. Coping suggestions for becoming accustomed to your hearing aids are also provided so that your experience out of the dispenser's office can be a successful one. Expectations for hearing amplified sound and using hearing aids are covered and a two-week program to help you ease into hearing aid use is offered.

Dispenser Adjustment of the Hearing Aid Controls

The dispenser adjusts the special options controls (see Chapter 9) on your hearing aids to achieve optimal correction of your hearing loss based on your listening comments and testing. The controls will be adjusted on the day you get the hearing aids and can be readjusted as needed at follow-up visits. Many dispensers have hearing aid test equipment and initially may adjust the hearing aids according to the electronic read-out of this equipment. Some hearing aids have no controls except the volume control and cannot be adjusted beyond the characteristics the manufacturer has built into them. The dispenser will have verified that the characteristics are appropriate for your hearing loss.

Adjusting hearing aid controls, however, requires more than reading charts and graphs. The way the hearing aids sound to you is important too. The dispenser will ask you questions about the sounds you hear while you are wearing the hearing aids. As the controls are adjusted, you will be asked to compare one sound to another. Your impressions of the sounds are used to set the hearing aid controls. Some of the questions the dispenser will ask (or you should volunteer information about) follow.

1. Does the dispenser's voice sound comfortably loud?

2. Does the dispenser's voice sound natural?

3. How does your own voice sound to you?

4. Does your own voice sound hollow or like you're speaking in a barrel?

5. Is sound tinny or sharp?

6. How do a variety of noises in the office (such as paper rustling, ventilation system, phone ringing, door slamming) sound?

New hearing aid users, who are not used to amplified sound, may find it difficult to answer these questions. The dispenser may have you use the hearing aids for one to two weeks and then ask you similar questions at follow-up visits. Further adjustments can be made after you have become more accustomed to amplified sound. Your answers to these questions guide the dispenser in adjusting your hearing aids. For example, a tinny sound or a hollow sound can usually be remedied by proper adjusting.

Aided Hearing Testing

It is important for the dispenser to verify that the settings of the hearing aids are appropriate and provide adequate correction of your hearing loss. If the correction is inadequate, then readjustment, fitting modifications (such as changing the shape of the earmold or ITE/ITC) or even different hearing aids may be indicated. While your subjective impressions are very important, other tests can be crucial as well. It is not uncommon for a new hearing aid user to report total satisfaction with a hearing aid, but testing fails to reveal measurable improvement. In this case the user may need more counseling about how to use the aid effectively. Or, the dispenser may need to readjust the hearing aid.

The most objective way to get such information is to test your hearing while you are wearing the hearing aids. This is called aided hearing testing.

Aided hearing testing is accomplished by two methods: functional gain and real-ear measurements. Either or both types of testing may be done. The functional gain method involves testing your hearing for tones (and often speech) both with and without wearing your hearing aids. Instead of using earphones, as in the initial hearing testing, the sounds are presented through loudspeakers. You again press a button or raise your hand when you hear the sounds and you may be asked to repeat words. The dispenser adjusts the hearing aid controls until the best correction of your loss is measured.

Real-ear measurements require special equipment in which a miniaturized microphone in a small plastic tube is inserted into your ear canal. The microphone measures the loudness of sounds presented through a loudspeaker both with and without the hearing aids. The dispenser adjusts the hearing aid controls to obtain the best hearing loss correction.

Setting Your Expectations for Hearing Aid Use

After the controls of the hearing aids have been properly adjusted, you need to wear them and begin getting accustomed to your new way of hearing. People derive different improvements in their hearing from hearing aids. Some notice a dramatic improvement; others notice subtle improvements. The improvement in hearing that you get partly depends on the amount of hearing loss you have, the situations you experience difficulty in, and your attitudes and expectations about wearing hearing aids. General statements apply to most hearing aid users, however, regardless of these factors. The following information may help set your expectations for hearing aid use and allow you to get maximum benefit from your aids.

1. *Wear your hearing aids as much as possible.* Since you have made the decision to try hearing aids, you need to give them a fair trial. And you need to wear them consis-

tently. The more you wear your hearing aids, the more successful you will be in using them effectively. If you only wear them once a week, to church, for example, you will never get used to how they feel in your ears, the sound of your own voice or the sound of amplification. Sounds will constantly startle you, and you will not be satisfied with the aids. Also, do not wear the hearing aids turned off in your ears. Then they function as ear plugs which doesn't help you get used to amplified sound and actually blocks sound from entering your ears. Always wear the hearing aids turned on!

You may ultimately decide that you only need or want to wear the hearing aids at certain times, but this decision should be based on actual wearing experience rather than the assumption that you don't need them. Try them everywhere, many times. You don't know what you're missing until you hear it again.

2. *Remember that hearing aids are an* aid *to hearing, not a cure for hearing loss.* Hearing aids definitely help you hear better. Despite the technological advances over the years, however, a hearing aid does not duplicate normal hearing. You hear speech and sounds better with hearing aids, but you still will experience difficulty understanding, or distinguishing, words in some situations. You will still need to ask for repetitions and you will still have some trouble sorting out words in noisy places. But, the hearing aids can be expected to relieve some of the stress of communication caused by having to listen so hard. You can expect to hear and understand better in many or most situations, but not in every one.

3. *Hearing aids do not block out all background noise, even with noise reduction circuits.* Regardless of what you read in the advertisements, hearing aids do not yet have the capability of eliminating background noise, leaving conversation crystal clear and easy to hear. Nor is any hearing aid smart enough to know which person's voice you are trying to hear out of a crowd. As discussed in Chapter 9, some hearing aids have noise reduction circuits which *reduce,* not eliminate, background noise.

4. *Hearing aids amplify the sound that is right around you.* Hearing aids will not pick up sounds much beyond 10 to 15 feet away from you, unless those sounds are quite loud. They pick up sounds best at 3 to 6 feet. That means you will hear better if you sit closer to what or whomever you are trying to hear. For example, it is best to sit near the front of the church and where you have a good view of the minister even when you wear hearing aids. If you sit too far away, you will miss out on the sermon and instead, hear people around you shuffling their feet and hymnals. This is also true if you attend meetings or lectures. Sit near the front whenever you can.

5. *Most hearing aids detect louder sounds better than softer sounds.* This is also true of our ears. It is easier to hear a person speaking in a conversational tone of voice than it is to hear someone whispering, even if you have normal hearing. Hearing aids pick up and amplify louder sounds, sometimes at the expense of softer sounds. This is why, at a restaurant for example, you may seem to hear the talking from surrounding, louder tables better than you can hear your own dinner companions who are talking more softly.

6. *Your hearing aid experience is a personal one.* You may know people who complain about their hearing aids and perhaps do not even wear them. You may also know other people who love their hearing aids. Try not to let another person's experience affect your own. You need to try hearing aids and adjust to them in your own way. If you need more time to adjust to them than your friend does, that doesn't mean you have failed or that you won't be successful. If you are more successful than a friend has been, perhaps you can encourage him or her to keep trying. Let your own experiences be your guide.

Returning the Hearing Aids

If you feel that you cannot adjust to using hearing aids or if you've decided you just don't want the hearing aids, you should return them. It is better to return them than to keep them in a drawer. Use the hearing aids for the whole trial period allotted and give them your best try. Remember that the return period and conditions are specified in your purchase agreement, so you must return the hearing aids according to that agreement. If you return them, that doesn't mean that you can't try hearing aids again in the future.

Before returning your hearing aids however, be sure that you've discussed all the problems with your dispenser. The dispenser can adjust and change controls and can even have you try different styles of hearing aids. Exhaust all the possibilities before returning them to be sure you've given yourself every opportunity to hear better.

A Two-Week Program for Beginning Your Adjustment to Hearing Aids

Hearing loss from aging typically progresses over the years. Over those years, you have adjusted to not hearing well. Now you must adjust to hearing again. You need to do this according to your own schedule because hearing loss and hearing again are different for each person. Often people are able to adjust to hearing aids within a few days, but many people also need longer to adjust.

At first, all sounds may seem to jump out at you and be equally noticeable. It takes practice and time to learn to listen again and to sort out important sounds from the less important ones. Eventually your brain learns to do this just as when you had normal hearing. For example, the refrigerator or furnace motor turning on may startle you at first, but after awhile you learn what that sound is and you pay less attention to it.

The following two-week program is offered to start you on the way to successful hearing aid use if you feel you are not adjusting in the first few days. Complete adjustment to hearing aids takes longer than two weeks. The eventual aim is to be able to wear your hearing aids all day. If you can do this right away, you should do so and feel very pleased. If you can't, it certainly doesn't mean you won't be able to in time. It means you'll have to work toward that goal and these suggestions may help you get going. If you are adjusting well after beginning this program, feel free to accelerate the steps as fits your needs and lifestyle.

The First Week

1. *Wear your hearing aids only at home for the first week, even if you are alone most of the time.*

2. *Wear the hearing aids each day for as long as you feel comfortable doing so.* Put them on in the morning, after you have washed or bathed, and see how long you can leave them on. It is as important to get used to the feeling of them in your ears as it is to get used to the way things sound through them. If you get tired or irritable after awhile, take them out and give yourself a break. If you can only wear the aids for an hour at a time in the beginning that's all right. Wait a couple of hours before trying them on again. Try to wear them for longer and longer periods, 3 to 4 times a day.

3. *Listen to the sounds in your home carefully and become accustomed to them.* Listen to the hum of the refrigerator, the furnace, air conditioner or fan. Notice if flourescent light bulbs make a hum or buzz. You may find that the telephone or door bell ringing are startling. Rustle newspapers and listen to their sharp crackle. Notice how dishes and silverware clang when you set the table or wash them. Turn the water faucet on and flush the toilet — these have been described as sounding like Niagara Falls by many people! While sitting quietly, just listen to the sounds your home makes.

4. *Read aloud to yourself and listen to the sound of your own voice.* It should sound louder than it normally does to you.

5. *Talk with only one person at a time, if possible, in a quiet room.* This is the easiest listening situation. It allows you to become accustomed to the sound of amplified speech

without any distractions. You can use each conversation with different individuals as a practice session. Some people speak clearly and are easy to understand. Other people really do mumble. It is important to get used to the speech and habits of different speakers and to get used to how the hearing aids help you hear them better. Some words may sound similar to you, for example, "carve" may sound like "car" or you might hear "egg" instead of "eggs." As discussed in Chapter 6, you can learn to tell the difference by the context of the conversation, watching the person talk, and learning to hear sound distinctions again. Improvements in hearing sound distinctions may take about eight weeks to begin to be noticeable, so don't get discouraged.

While you are talking with each person, also practice moving the volume control softer and louder to discover which setting lets you hear that person the best without straining.

6. *Listen to a favorite television or radio program each day while wearing your hearing aids.* Voices on TV and radio are amplified already and may sound different through your hearing aids. The aids may improve the clarity of the voices as you practice listening with them.

The Second Week

1. *Continue practicing items 2 through 6 in the First Week program, but do them for longer periods of time.*

2. *Wear the hearing aids for as many hours as you comfortably are able to.* Ideally, you should be able to wear the hearing aids all day without being very aware of them in

your ears. It is especially important to wear them all day, if possible, during your trial period so that you can learn when the aids are beneficial and when, if ever, they are not. The trial period is the time to decide whether or not you will keep the hearing aids. You can't make this decision if you don't wear them consistently. Even if you are alone most of the day, wear them anyway, and continue getting used to them.

3. *Wear the hearing aids outside and listen to the sounds around you.* Take a short walk and try to identify birds singing, traffic sounds, rustling leaves, and other sounds you encounter. On a windy day, your hearing aids may amplify wind noise, and it will sound like you're in a wind tunnel. This can be an annoying sound. If you're caught on a windy day and it bothers you, turn the hearing aids down or even take them out. Tell your dispenser about bothersome wind noise because special screens and hoods can be added to your aids to reduce this problem.

4. *Talk with, and practice listening to, more than one person at a time, in a quiet setting.* It takes practice to distinguish one person's voice from another's while keeping up with the conversation. Do this step each day. Remember to cue into the context of the conversation and to watch people as they talk. If you have trouble, ask them to repeat. Adjust the volume of the hearing aids so the voices are easily and comfortably heard.

5. *Converse with one or more persons in a slightly noisy place.* You can go somewhere noisier than your home or you can add your own background noise at home. For example, turn the TV or radio on so that you can hear it, though not too loudly. Ordinarily you wouldn't want to deliberately

interfere with communication, but this is for you to practice listening in background noise. You will encounter similar situations, and it will help if you have practiced.

Begin this step by just talking with one person and, when you feel that you have practiced enough, add more people to your group. This can be made into a social gathering and no one will even know that you are practicing using your hearing aids. Practicing this step does not end with Week 2, but continues until you feel confident.

6. *Begin wearing your hearing aids in public places.* This step should begin in the second week and continue until you have experienced wearing your hearing aids in most of the situations you are commonly in. Start by going to a lecture or church or even a music concert. If there is not a raised podium or stage, sit in the first or second row. If there is a raised podium or stage, sit a few rows back from the front so you don't have to look up. Adjust the volume of the hearing aids so that you can hear comfortably. Sudden loud sounds, like clapping or the organ starting to play, will be loud in comparison to the speaker's voice and you may need to turn the aids down then.

Gradually expose yourself to louder, noisier situations. Wear your hearing aids to the grocery store or shopping mall and finally wear them to restaurants, dining halls, and large social gatherings. Practicing this step can easily be combined with Step 5, discussed previously.

Voices in large groups may still seem like a jumble and background noise can cover up the person you are trying to hear. Adjust the volume a bit lower (softer) to the point where the noise is less noticeable but the voices around you are still slightly louder. This will be difficult at first. It takes practice to be able to adjust your volume quickly and to learn to tune out some background noise, all the while following the conversation. These situations may also try your patience. If you have trouble in one situation, do not give up. Continue to use your hearing aids in all places for at least part of the time you are there. If you need to, you can always take them out for awhile, but this should be your final action. Before taking the aids off, try reducing the volume systematically, even if it is very low.

With continued practice and perseverance, you will start to notice that you can wear your hearing aids in most situations and be successful in hearing better. This may take a week or a month and it may take a year or more; everyone is different. The important thing is to keep at it.

Chapter 13

Hearing Aid Repairs

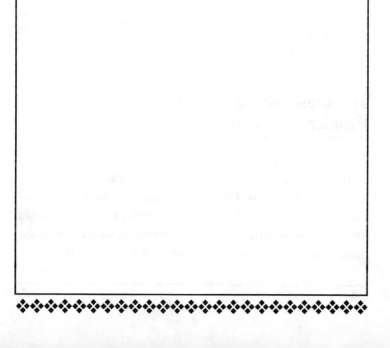

Hearing aids are subjected to long hours of use each day, many more hours than you drive your car, operate an oven, or even have your television turned on. They are small, relatively delicate electronic devices and they will sometimes malfunction. Given their daily exposure to humidity, sweat, earwax, and skin oils, it's surprising they don't malfunction more often. Sometimes the problem with your hearing aids is something simple that you can troubleshoot yourself and fix at home. If that doesn't work, your hearing aid dispenser may be able to fix them for you. Sometimes the dispenser must send your hearing aids to the manufacturer for repair.

This chapter outlines steps to try at home when your hearing aids malfunction, which may save you a trip to the dispenser's office. These malfunctions include no sound or weak sound, cutting on and off, and constant squealing. Repairs that are done by the dispenser and the manufacturer are also explained, including in-warranty and out-of-warranty repairs. You may be able to use a loaner hearing aid while yours are being repaired and this is reviewed at the end of the chapter.

Troubleshooting Your Hearing Aid Problems at Home

Some day, it's going to happen. You turn on one of your hearing aids and there is no sound. Or the sound is very weak and distorted. Or maybe it just squeals and won't stop. You don't need to call your hearing aid dispenser until you first rule out some common causes of these problems — some of which you can fix yourself.

Problem 1: Hearing Aid is Dead or Weak

Several causes of these symptoms may have nothing to do with the internal wiring or parts. Check these causes first:

1. *Dead Battery.* Try a new battery. If it still doesn't work, try a battery from another package. It is possible to get a bad pack of batteries so it helps to try one from a different package. You could also invest a few dollars in a button-cell battery tester so you can test your batteries. Battery testers are available at hardware stores, electronic parts stores, and usually from your hearing aid dispenser.

2. *Battery is inverted.* On some hearing aids, it is possible to close the battery door even when the battery is put in upside down. The hearing aid will not operate with the battery upside down, so check to see that you've put it in correctly. If you have jammed the battery inside the aid, don't force the door open because it may break. Take it to your dispenser if you can't get the battery out. If the door does break, however, don't worry because doors are easily replaced.

3. *Hearing aid or earmold holes are plugged with earwax or debris.* Gently use a wax pick/loop or a brush (see illustration on page 149) on an ITE, ITC, or earmold to pick wax and debris out of the openings. *Do not* jam the wax farther inside, just pick it out. ITEs and ITCs have a plastic tubing inside of one of the openings. Do not attempt to pull or pick the tubing out. The tubing is usually clear or flesh colored and is often mistaken for debris.

Remember that the earmold can be disconnected from a BTE or eyeglass hearing aid for cleaning. Review Chapter 11 and the illustration on page 151 for instructions.

4. *The hearing aid is damp or wet.* This can be caused by accidents like wearing it in the shower or swimming pool, by washing it in the washing machine or by things you wouldn't necessarily think of, like sweating or high humidity. Any moisture can cause a hearing aid to be dead (no sound) or to sound weak and distorted.

If you suspect moisture, dry the hearing aid off with a tissue. Take the battery out and leave the hearing aid in a dry place overnight. Then try it again the next morning. Do not attempt to dry a hearing aid by putting it under a lamp or in direct sunlight. Do not dry it off with a hair dryer or bake the moisture out in a microwave or regular oven.

You can purchase a drying kit from your dispenser, and this is recommended if you perspire a lot or if you live in a humid part of the country. Drying kits are inexpensive, reusable jars filled with a drying agent. You should keep your hearing aids in it every night, but be sure to take the batteries out first.

5. *The switch is in the wrong position.* If your hearing aid has a telecoil (T) switch, an ON-OFF switch or a noise suppression switch, make sure the switch is in the ON position. If the switch is accidentally turned to either the telecoil or the OFF position, for example, you will not hear anything. Switch position is easy to check on a BTE or eyeglass hearing aid because the positions are usually marked with letters. Remember that "M" (or letters like "L", "N" or "H") is ON while "O" is OFF. If the positions on your hearing aid are not labeled (they are not on ITEs or ITCs), hold the hearing aid cupped in your hand with the volume turned up. Move the switch back and forth

and listen for the squeal. When you hear the squeal, the aid is ON.

Problem 2: Hearing Aid Cuts On and Off or Fades

This problem often signals a short in the hearing aid or a problem with the components or battery contacts. However, there are a couple of things you should check before taking the aid to the dispenser.

1. *Battery is weak or dying.* Again, try a new battery or batteries. A new battery will resolve the problem if that was the cause.

2. *Hearing aid or earmold holes are plugged with wax.* See Number 2 under Problem 1.

3. *Earmold tubing is crimped.* (This does not apply to ITE or ITC aids.) This happens by squeezing the tubing when putting the earmold on or taking it off, or by twisting it when putting a BTE aid over the ear. Try to uncrimp the tube and see if the sound returns. If uncrimping the tubing does not restore sound, the tube may need to be replaced by the dispenser or there may be some problem with the aid.

Problem 3: Hearing Aid Squeals Constantly

This condition, called feedback, is sometimes caused by internal component problems (called internal feedback), but it is more often the result of a simple problem which you can figure out on your own.

1. *Hearing aid or earmold is not properly inserted in your ear.* If you don't put the hearing aid or earmold into your ear properly, it will squeal incessantly and may even fall out of your ear. Feel it in your ear and check the insertion in a mirror. See Chapter 11 and the illustrations on pages 135, 136, and 137 to review proper hearing aid and earmold insertion.

2. *The volume is turned too high (loud).* Try turning the volume down until the squeal disappears. If you have to turn the aid off or nearly off for the squeal to go away, the feedback is being caused by something else.

3. *Your ear canal is blocked by wax.* If earwax builds up in your ear canal, it causes the amplified sound coming out of the hearing aid to bounce off it and to leak back out of your ear. Then it is reamplified and feeds back, or squeals. Suspect earwax build-up if your hearing aid is frequently blocked by wax and if you have to clean the wax off nearly every time you take it out of your ear. If you suspect this is causing the problem, you need someone to examine your ears, preferably your physician or hearing aid dispenser, to see if wax is present. The wax should be removed by the physician. You should not try to remove it yourself because you can injure your ear. Some people produce more earwax than others. If you know you tend to have a wax build-up problem, have your ears cleaned regularly.

4. *Earmold tubing and/or earhook is broken* (does not apply to ITE or ITC aids). Earmold tubing needs to be replaced when it hardens and yellows, otherwise it may break or tiny cracks may develop. Replacement needs to be done once a year, sometimes more often. Earhooks on BTEs may break when the earmold tubing is disconnected from them.

Both are problems the dispenser can fix easily, so you'll need to take the hearing aid in.

5. *Hearing aid or earmold is too small.* A fitting problem such as this requires a trip to the dispenser, but you may be able to judge whether the fit is too loose. A hearing aid or earmold that is too small allows sound to leak back out of your ear and be reamplified. This results in feedback. Earmolds also can shrink with time and exposure to skin oils and acids. They need to be replaced periodically. If you have recently lost weight, your ear canal may become larger (less fat!) and the hearing aid or earmold will be too small. Finally, the hearing aid may have been made too small when it was manufactured. In all of these cases, the dispenser must check the fit and, if necessary, have it remade.

Caution

You should never open the case of the hearing aid or take it apart or attempt to repair or replace the components yourself. This usually results in greater damage to your hearing aid. Self-repair also negates your warranty, and the manufacturer will charge you for the repair.

Repairs Done by the Hearing Aid Dispenser

Some of the problems listed in the previous section will obviously need the attention of your hearing aid dispenser. The dispenser can do minor repairs in the office and you will get your hearing aid back right away. Hearing aid dispensers should be able to do the following repairs:

1. *Clean wax from the receiver.* If you have tried to remove it but didn't get it all out or if it's been pushed inside, the dispenser can do a more thorough and careful cleaning job. Some dispensers even use a microscope to look inside the receiver of your hearing aid to make sure it is completely cleaned out. If the tubing around the receiver is damaged by aggressive cleaning with a wax loop, some dispensers can replace it in the office. More often, though, damaged receiver tubing must be replaced by the manufacturer.

2. *Clean the battery contacts and adjust them.* Sometimes corrosion or rust develops in the battery compartment and on the contacts from moisture exposure. Your dispenser has special cleaning agents to remove it. The position of the contacts also can be adjusted for better battery contact if they are not in proper alignment.

3. *Clean the internal components.* Your dispenser may be able to partially disassemble the hearing aid to clean it internally with special sprays if it is very dirty. If your hearing aid is still under warranty, the dispenser usually won't do this as the warranty could be negated. Never attempt this on your own.

4. *Dry the hearing aid.* For hearing aids suspected to have moisture damage, the dispenser can put your hearing aid in a special drying kit for 24 to 48 hours. Sometimes this restores normal function. You can also purchase these kits from the dispenser to use at home.

5. *Reglue the hearing aid.* If your hearing aid has become unglued, the dispenser should have the correct glue to put it back together again. *Do not* glue a hearing aid together yourself. Remember, self-repair means that the manufacturer will not honor the warranty.

6. *Replace some parts, such as earmold tubing, earhooks, battery doors, volume control caps, and microphone or wind screens.* If a part comes off your hearing aid or breaks, call your dispenser. Most dispensers keep replacement parts on hand, and he or she may be able to put on a new part quickly and easily.

7. *Grind and buff the hearing aid or earmold to make it more comfortable or to reshape it as needed.* Your dispenser should be able to take care of minor fitting problems in the office. In some cases, however, the hearing aid or the earmold will have to be remade. Your dispenser can judge whether or not the aid or earmold must be remade.

After the dispenser determines the cause of the malfunction and repairs it, if possible, he or she will do a listening check on your hearing aid and may run it on test equipment, also called an electroacoustic check. An electroacoustic check allows the dispenser to compare the power, the gain (similar to volume), the frequency response (amplification of pitches), and the battery drain of your hearing aid to the manufacturer's specifications. They should match up. If they do not, the dispenser may have to send your aid to the manufacturer for repair.

What You Should Know About Warranty Repairs

Your hearing aid is guaranteed to be free of manufacturing defects for a given amount of time (usually one year) after purchase. The FDA requires manufacturers to provide a one-year warranty period on all new hearing aids, and that warranty is supposed to be passed along to the dispenser and the consumer. Some dispensers may not tell you that a warranty comes with the hearing aid, or they may charge you extra for even the one-year warranty. Consider comparison shopping before purchasing hearing aids from such a dispenser. Most dispensers offer a one-year warranty, and sometimes a longer one, at no extra charge. Most manufacturers also offer an extended warranty for repair (and sometimes replacement if the aid is lost) at the time of purchase. If you are interested in an extended warranty, ask your dispenser about purchasing one.

The manufacturer will fix most problems that arise during the warranty period (including remaking ITE and ITC aids) at no charge to the dispenser or to you. Your warranty period should be clearly stated on the purchase agreement, and it should be explained to you at the time of purchase. Technically, you should be able to take your hearing aid to any dispenser who deals with the manufacturer of your aid for a warranty repair, even if you did not purchase it from that dispenser. You may be charged a shipping or handling fee if you take it to a different dispenser, however.

The manufacturer reserves the right to cancel your warranty or to charge you for a repair if the problem with your aid is felt to be from abuse. Abuse can include repairing it yourself, smashing it to pieces (unintentionally), letting your pet chew on it, or damaging it from excessive exposure to heat or moisture.

Expect your hearing aid to be gone for one to two weeks when it is sent to the manufacturer for repair. Major manufacturers send repaired hearing aids back by two-day express mail and this speeds up the return time. Most manufacturers also offer one-day service and overnight return for an extra fee. If you need your aid within three to four days, ask the dispenser to arrange this quicker service.

What You Should Know About Out-of-Warranty Repairs

Once your hearing aid is out of the manufacturer's warranty period, it can still be repaired but you will be charged. A hearing aid is usually worth repairing for five years, unless it has needed so many repairs in that time that it is more cost effective to buy a new one. With proper care and maintenance, a hearing aid may last many years beyond five. Out-of-warranty repairs take as long as in-warranty repairs, about one to two weeks.

Hearing aid manufacturers guarantee the repair for a given period of time as part of the out-of-warranty repair charge. They usually provide a six-month warranty for hearing aids that are less than five years old. Some manufacturers also offer a 12-month warranty for an extra charge. Any repair problem, except for abuse, that arises during that time is covered by the charge.

Manufacturers prefer for you to buy a new hearing aid after five years. For this reason, some do not repair aids more than five years old. Those that do repair older hearing aids may charge more and only guarantee the repair for 30 to 90 days. There are hearing aid repair centers that repair all makes of older hearing aids and will provide longer repair warranty coverage. All-make repair centers do not necessarily use the specific manufacturer's parts, but this doesn't always matter. If your hearing aid is more than five years old and you feel it is worth repairing, an all-make repair center may be your only option. Your dispenser can send it to such a place.

Out-of-warranty repairs are a steady source of income for dispensers, and they all mark up the manufacturer's charge by varying amounts. In 1992, you could expect to pay $100.00 or more for a six-month repair warranty. If a dispenser tells you that there is no repair warranty period and still charges you that price, take your hearing aid somewhere else. *Some* warranty period is always provided by the manufacturer to the dispenser and you are entitled to it. You should feel free to call other dispensers in your area to compare repair charges and warranties. You do not have to have your hearing aid repaired by the dispenser you purchased it from, so you can shop around for the best price and services.

When considering an out-of-warranty hearing aid repair, ask the following questions:

1. What is the charge for a 6-month and a 12-month repair warranty?

2. Will the aid be sent to the manufacturer for repair or to an all-make repair center?

3. What is the repair warranty and charge from the manufacturer versus an all-make repair center (for hearing aids over five years of age)?

4. How long will the hearing aid be gone?

5. Can I use a loaner hearing aid while mine is being repaired?

Loaner Hearing Aids

If it is sent to the manufacturer, your hearing aid will be gone for one to two weeks. During that time you will be without a hearing aid, unless you usually wear two, own a spare one or ask for a loaner. If you wear two hearing aids and only one needs repair, you can usually get by with your other aid.

Most dispensers have BTE hearing aids available to loan. Loaners are often older hearing aids that have been donated by clients or reconditioned by manufacturers. They are rarely the same model that you wear, but they will still work for you. Recall that BTE and eyeglass hearing aids require an earmold to fit in your ear. If you usually wear one of these aids or if you have your own earmold, you will be able to use a loaner hearing aid.

Because ITE and ITC hearing aids have no earmolds and are made specifically for your ear, you probably will not be given an ITE or ITC loaner. Occasionally dispensers have "one size fits all" premolded ITE and ITC aids for sale or for loan or have old, donated ITE aids available, but do not count on this. More commonly, dispensers have stock earmolds which are produced in general sizes and shapes. A stock earmold may fit your ear fairly well but probably not exactly. The dispenser may be able to modify a stock earmold for better fit so that you can borrow a BTE loaner aid. A wise investment is to have an earmold made for yourself to use in the event of a repair. Most people don't think of this until their hearing aid is sent for repair, but an earmold can be made at any time at a small charge. If you do this in advance, you will be prepared. Often, people who have an ITE or ITC aid that is sent for repair, just do without until their hearing aid comes back. That can be a very long one to two weeks.

Taking care of your hearing aids each day and returning to your dispenser for a yearly check and cleaning will cut down on repair problems. Eventually though, regardless of how careful you are, most hearing aids will need attention. If it is a problem you can't solve yourself by following the troubleshooting instructions in this chapter, take it to your dispenser. Hearing aids can be fixed.

Chapter 14

Sources for Additional Information

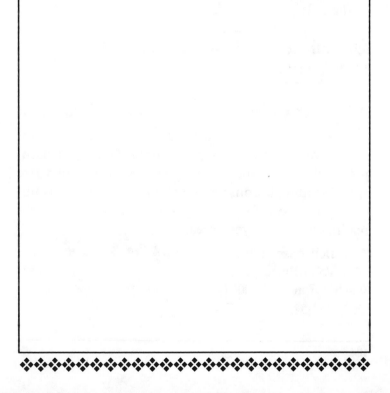

Many organizations, institutions, and associations publish excellent information about hearing loss, hearing instruments, and hearing help. Some organizations can be joined and even have local chapter meetings and national conventions. If you are interested in pursuing any of the topics you have read about in this book in greater detail, a list of recommended sources is provided. The list is not exhaustive but offers a representative sample.

A short list of companies that sell products of interest to people with hearing loss is provided at the end of this chapter. Catalogs from these companies have helpful gadgets such as loud smoke alarms, door bells, and alarm clocks, among others, and listening devices for televisions and telephones. These products make practical and interesting gifts too.

Organizations, Institutions, and Associations

Alexander Graham Bell Association for the Deaf

This organization provides educational materials for people who are hearing impaired or deaf and has a list of publications available. They also maintain a list of where speechreading lessons can be obtained across the country. Write or call for a listing of titles or to find speechreading lessons in your area.

A.G. Bell Association
3417 Volta Place, N.W.
Washington, DC 20007
(202) 337-5220

American Academy of Audiology (AAA)

AAA is a professional organization that is establishing educational guidelines and requirements for audiologists, and guidelines for the profession in general. Contact AAA for more information about audiology, hearing loss, and hearing help.

AAA
c/o Dr. Northern
University of Colorado Health Science Center
P.O. Box 210
4200 E. 9th Street
Denver, CO 80262
(303) 394-7856

American Academy of Otolaryngology (AAO)

This organization represents ENT physicians in government and regulates their medical education. They have a listing of publication titles available that cover ear problems, ear care, and hearing. They also can help you find ENT services in your area.

AAO
1101 Vermont Ave., N.W., Suite 302
Washington, DC 20005
(703) 836-4444

American Association for Retired Persons (AARP)

AARP has published two very helpful brochures, among others, called *Have You Heard? Hearing Loss and Aging*

(Catalog No. D12219) and *Product Report: Hearing Aids* (Catalog No. D13766). They can be ordered by written request, and you also can request a complete list of their publications.

AARP Fulfillment
1909 K Street, N.W.
Washington, DC 20049

American Speech-Language-Hearing Association (ASHA)

This is the professional organization that certifies audiologists (and speech-language pathologists) and regulates their education. ASHA has a toll-free consumer helpline you can call, or you can write to them for a list of pamphlet and book titles about audiologists, hearing loss, hearing instruments, and audiology services in your area.

ASHA
10801 Rockville Pike
Rockville, MD 20852
Consumer Helpline: (800) 638-8255
(in Maryland: (301) 897-8682)

Better Hearing Institute (BHI)

BHI is a consumer-oriented educational organization that publishes information about current medical and technological progress in dealing with hearing loss. Call them toll-free.

BHI
P.O. Box 1840
Washington, DC 20013
(800) EAR-WELL

Food and Drug Administration (FDA)

This government agency provides information pamphlets about hearing and hearing aids.

FDA Office of Consumer Affairs
5600 Fishers Lane
Rockville, MD 20857
(301) 443-3170

House Ear Institute

This medical facility conducts clinical ear and hearing research and performs ear surgery. Information about ear problems, hearing loss, hearing aids, cochlear implants, and other medical treatment is available by writing or calling.

House Ear Institute
256 South Lake Street
Los Angeles, CA 90057
(213) 483-4431

National Button Battery Hotline

Call this telephone number immediately if you or someone else has swallowed a hearing aid battery. They will recommend the appropriate treatment, and they expect you — or your doctor — to call collect.

Call Collect: (202) 625-3333

National Council of Senior Citizens

This group is dedicated to advocacy of senior citizen health and housing issues. You may write to them or call for information about these topics and for membership information.

National Council of Senior Citizens
1331 F Street, N.W.
Washington, DC 20004
(202) 347-8800

National Hearing Aid Society (NHAS)

This is the professional organization of hearing aid dispensers which oversees certification for hearing instrument specialists. Call the toll-free consumer helpline or write for information about hearing loss and hearing help. They can provide the names of hearing aid dispensers in your area.

NHAS
20361 Middlebelt Road
Livonia, MI 48152
Consumer Helpline: (800) 521-5247

National Information Center on Deafness (NICD)

NICD is an information center at Gallaudet University. They have a complete listing of most organizations and institutions, along with publication titles available from each organization and prices. Call or write to request a copy of this comprehensive list.

NICD
Gallaudet University
800 Florida Avenue, N.E.
Washington, DC 20002
(202) 651-5051

New York League for the Hard of Hearing

This is a non-profit agency for rehabilitation of hearing loss in children and adults. Audiologists test hearing and fit hearing aids at their offices. They have a wealth of public information available and they publish the Hearing Rehabilitation Quarterly. Write to request a listing of titles or to find out about obtaining hearing aids if you live in that area.

New York League for the Hard of Hearing
71 West 23rd Street
New York, NY 10010
(212) 741-7650

Self Help for Hard of Hearing People (SHHH)

SHHH is a national organization of people who are hearing impaired. There are state and local chapters. They promote awareness of and information about hearing loss, communication, and hearing instruments. They publish a quarterly journal, *SHHH Journal,* and have an annual national convention. Contact the national office to find out whether there is a local group in your area or to join the national group. You may also request information about their publications.

SHHH
7800 Wisconsin Avenue
Bethesda, MD 20814
(301) 657-2248

Product Information

The following companies can be contacted for a catalogue or for product information. This is not a complete list of companies that sell products for people with hearing loss. Your hearing aid dispenser may know of others.

AT&T

AT&T has a special needs department to address the product needs of people who are hearing impaired. They sell amplifier phones, phones with loud bells, and listening devices. You may write or call for a copy of their product information.

AT&T National Special Needs Center
2001 Route 46, Suite 310
Parsippany, NJ 07054-9990
(800) 233-1222

HARC Mercantile, Inc.

HARC Mercantile has a catalog of products made for people who are hearing impaired. Items include alerting systems, smoke alarms, loud telephones and doorbells, and a host of other products.

HARC Mercantile, Inc.
P.O. Box 3055
Kalamazoo, MI 49003-3055
(800) 445-9968 (U.S.)
(800) 962-6634 (MI)

National Captioning Institute (NCI)

The National Captioning Institute has information about and sells the decoding devices for closed-captioned television programs. You may think this is only for "deaf" people but those with any amount of hearing loss can use them. Many TV shows are now closed captioned, and you may find it easier to read along with a program rather than trying to listen and understand all that is being spoken.

NCI
5203 Leesburg Pike
Falls Church, VA 22041

Radio Shack

Radio Shack sells special listening devices for televisions and telephones and other items. Write for their free catalog.

Radio Shack Special Needs Catalog
Department 88-A-393
300 1 Tandy Center
Ft. Worth, TX 76102

Your Local Telephone Company

Local telephone companies and telephone stores have amplifier phones, and phones with loud bells available for people with hearing loss. Look in the information section of your telephone book for the toll-free number under Special Needs or Handicapped Services.

Your Local Hospital or Medical Clinic Department of Audiology or Department of Speech and Hearing

If you are looking for a specific product or some help in finding out what products are available for people with hearing loss, your local audiologist should be able to guide you to the correct companies or catalogs.

Appendix A

State Licensing Agencies for Audiologists

Alabama
Alabama Board of Examiners
for Speech Pathology and
Audiology
555 South Perry Street
P.O. Box 20833
Montgomery, AL 36120-0833
(205) 834-2415

Alaska
Division of Occupational
Licensing
P.O. Box D
Juneau, AK 99811-0800

Arkansas
Arkansas Board of Examiners
for Speech Pathology and
Audiology
P.O. Box 25035
Little Rock, AR 72225-0345
(501) 371-6070

California
Speech Pathology and
Audiology Examining
Committee
Board of Medical Quality
Assurance
1430 Howe Avenue
Sacramento, CA 95825
(916) 920-6388

Connecticut
Speech Pathology and
Audiology Licensing
Department of Health Services
Division of Medical Quality
Assurance
150 Washington Street

Hartford, CT 06106
(203) 566-1039

Delaware
Board of Audiologists, Speech
Pathologists and Hearing Aid
Dispensers
Office of Professional Licensing
O'Neill Building, P.O. Box 1401
Dover, DE 19903
(302) 736-4522

Florida
Board of Speech-Language
Pathology and Audiology
Department of Professional
Regulation
Northwood Center
1940 North Monroe Street
Tallahassee, FL 32399-0782
(904) 487-3041

Georgia
Georgia Board of Examiners
for Speech Pathology and
Audiology
166 Pryor Street, S.W.
Atlanta, GA 30303
(404) 656-6719

Hawaii
Speech Pathology and
Audiology Board of Examiners
Department of Commerce and
Consumer Affairs
1010 Richard Street
Honolulu, HI 96813
(808) 548-8542

Illinois
Board of Speech-Language
Pathologists and Audiologists

Source: List reprinted with permission from the American Speech-Language-Hearing Association. *Asha, 22* (3), 113.

Department of Professional
  Regulation
320 West Washington
Springfield, IL 62704
(217) 785-0800

Indiana
Indiana Speech-Language
Pathology and Audiology
Board
One American Square
Suite 1020, Box 82067
Indianapolis, IN 46282
(317) 232-2960

Iowa
Iowa State Board of Speech
  Pathology and Audiology
  Examiners
State Department of Health
Lucas State Office Building
Des Moines, IA 50319-0075
(515) 281-4408

Kentucky
Board of Examiners of Speech
  Pathologists and Audiologists
P.O. Box 456
Frankfort, KY 40602
(502) 564-3296

Louisiana
Louisiana Board of Examiners
  for Speech Pathology and
  Audiology
P.O. Box 355
Prairieville, LA 70769
(504) 673-3139

Maine
Board of Examiners of Speech
  Pathology and Audiology

Division of Licensing and
  Enforcement
State House Station 35
Augusta, ME 04333
(207) 582-8723

Maryland
Boards of Examiners for
  Speech Pathologists and
  Audiologists
4201 Patterson Avenue, Third
  Floor
Baltimore, MD 21215-2299
(301) 764-4725

Massachusetts
Board of Registration for
  Speech-Language Pathology
  and Audiology
Division of Registration
100 Cambridge Street, 15th Floor
Boston, MA 02202
(617) 727-1747

Mississippi
Mississippi Council of Advisors
  in Speech Pathology and
  Audiology
Mississippi State Department
  of Health
P.O. Box 1700-2423 North
  State Street
Jackson, MS 39215-1700
(601) 960-7504

Missouri
Missouri Committee of Speech
  Pathology and Clinical
  Audiology
P.O. Box 4
Jefferson City, MO 65102
(314) 751-0098

Montana
Board of Speech Pathologists
and Audiologists
Bureau of Professional Licensing
111 North Jackson, Arcade
Building
Helena, MT 59620-0407
(406) 444-4282

Nebraska
Board of Examiners in
Audiology and Speech
Pathology
Bureau of Examining Boards
Department of Health
P.O. Box 95007
Lincoln, NE 68509-5007
(402) 471-2115

Nevada
Nevada Board of Examiners for
Audiology and Speech
Pathology
Department of Speech
Pathology and Audiology
University of Nevada School of
Medicine
Reno, NV 89557-0046
(702) 784-4887

New Jersey
Audiology and Speech-Language
Pathology Advisory Committee
NJ Division of Consumer
Affairs
1100 Raymond Boulevard,
Room 507
Newark, NJ 07102
(201) 648-3571

New Mexico
Speech-Language Pathology
and Audiology Advisory Board

Boards and Commissions
Division
Regulation and Licensing
Department
P.O. Box 25101
Santa Fe, NM 87504-1388
(505) 827-7164

New York
Speech Pathology and Audiology
Unit
State Education Department
Cultural Education Center,
Room 3025
Albany, NY 12230
(518) 486-6059

North Carolina
Board of Examiners for Speech
and Language Pathologists
and Audiologists
P.O. Box 5545
Greensboro, NC 27403
(919) 272-1828

North Dakota
Board of Examiners on
Audiology and Speech-
Language Pathology
Box 8158 UND
Grand Forks, ND 58202-8158
(707) 777-4421

Ohio
Board of Speech Pathology and
Audiology
77 South High Street, 16th Floor
Columbus, OH 43266
(614) 466-3145

Oklahoma
State Board of Examiners for
Speech Pathology and
Audiology

P.O. Box 53592
State Capital Station
Oklahoma City, OK 73152
(405) 521-6131

Oregon
Board of Examiners for Speech
  Pathology and Audiology
1400 Southwest Fifth Avenue
Portland, OR 97201
(503) 229-5390

Pennsylvania
State Board of Examiners in
  Speech-Language Pathology,
  Audiology, and Teachers of
  the Hearing Impaired
Bureau of Professional and
  Occupational Affairs
P.O. Box 2649
Harrisburg, PA 17105-2649
(717) 783-7156

Rhode Island
State Board of Examiners for
  Speech Pathology and
  Audiology
Department of Professional
  Regulation
Cannon Building
3 Capital Hill, Room H104
Providence, RI 02908
(401) 277-2827

South Carolina
South Carolina Board of
  Examiners in Speech
  Pathology and Audiology
P.O. Box 11876
Columbia, SC 29211
(803) 772-0260

Tennessee
State Board of Examiners for
  Speech Pathology and
  Audiology
Department of Public Health
283 Plus Park Boulevard
Nashville, TN 37219
(615) 367-6243

Texas
State Committee of Examiners
  for Speech-Language
  Pathology and Audiology
1100 West 49th Street
Austin, TX 78756-3183
(512) 459-2935

Utah
Speech Pathology and
  Audiology Advisory Board
Division of Occupational and
  Professional Licensing
160 East 300 South
P.O. Box 45802
Salt Lake City, UT 84145
(801) 530-6628

Virginia
State Board of Examiners for
  Audiology and Speech
  Pathology
Department of Health
  Regulatory Boards
1601 Rolling Hills Drive
Richmond, VA 23229-5005
(804) 662-9111

Wisconsin
Council on Speech-Language
  Pathology and Audiology
Department of Regulation and
  Licensing

Bureau of Health Professions
P.O. Box 8935
Madison, WI 53708-8935
(608) 267-9377

Wyoming
State Board of Examiners in
  Speech Pathology and
  Audiology
2008 Gregg Avenue
Worlund, WY 82401
(307) 347-2435

Appendix **B**

Regulatory Agencies for Hearing Aid Specialists

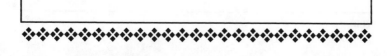

Alabama
Hearing Aid Board
State Health Department
328 State Office Building
Montgomery, AL 36130
(205) 261-5004

Alaska
Department of Commerce and
Economic Development
Division of Occupational
Licensure-Hearing Aid
Dealers and Audiologists
P.O. Box D-LIC
Juneau, AK 99811-0800
(907) 465-2541

Arizona
Hearing Conservation Program
Department of Health Services
1740 West Adams, Room 212
Phoenix, AZ 85007
(602) 255-1181

Arkansas
Arkansas Board of H.A.
Dispensers
#10 Corporate Hill Drive
Suite 350
Little Rock, AR 72205
(501) 228-9888

California
Dispensers Examining
Committee
1430 Howe Avenue
Suite 52
Sacramento, CA 95825
(916) 920-6377

Colorado
No regulation

Connecticut
Hearing Aid Dealers Licensing
Board
Department of Health Services
Division of Medical Quality
Assurance
150 Washington Street
Hartford, CT 06106
(203) 566-1039

Delaware
Advisory Council on Hearing
Aids
Division of Public Health
O'Neill Building
P.O. Box 1401
Dover, DE 19903
(302) 736-4796

District of Columbia
Department of Consumer and
Regulatory Affairs
Division of Pharmaceutical and
Medical Devices Control
614 H Street, N.W., Room 1016
Washington, DC 20013
(202) 727-7219

Florida
Board of Hearing Aid
Specialists
130 North Monroe Street
Tallahassee, FL 32301
(904) 487-1813

Georgia
Board of Hearing Aid Dealers
and Dispensers

Source: List reprinted with permission from the American Speech-Language-Hearing Association. 1991. *Asha, 22*(3), p. 115–116.

166 Pryor Street, S.W.
Atlanta, GA 30303
(404) 656-3912

Hawaii
Board of Hearing Aid Dealers
and Fitters
Department of Commerce and
Consumer Affairs
Professional and Vocational
Licensing Division
P.O. Box 3469
Honolulu, HI 96801
(808) 548-4100

Idaho
Hearing Aid Dealers and
Fitters
Bureau of Occupational
Licensing
2417 Bank Drive
Boise, ID 83705
(208) 334-3233

Illinois
Hearing Aid Consumer
Protection Program
Department of Public Health
Division of Health Assessment
and Screening
535 West Jefferson
Springfield, IL 62761
(217) 782-4733

Indiana
Hearing Aid Dealers Advisory
Committee
Health Professions Service
Bureau
One American Square
Suite 1020, Box 82067

Indianapolis, IN 46282
(317) 232-2960

Iowa
Board of Examiners for the
Licensing and Regulation of
Hearing Aid Dealers
State Department of Health
Lucas State Office Building
Des Moines, IA 50317
(515) 281-4408

Kansas
Kansas Board of Hearing Aids
P.O. Box 252
Wichita, KS 67201
(316) 263-0774

Kentucky
Board of Licensing Hearing
Aid Dealers
P.O. Box 456
Frankfort, KY 40602
(502) 564-3296

Louisiana
State Board of Hearing Aid
Dealers
P.O. Box 499
Baton Rouge, LA 70821
(504) 344-5828

Maine
Board of Hearing Aid Dealers
and Fitters
Division of Licensing and
Enforcement
State House Station 35
Augusta, ME 04333
(207) 289-3671

Maryland
Board of Examiners for
  Hearing Aid Dealers
501 St. Paul Place, Room 902
Baltimore, MD 21201
(301) 333-6322

Massachusetts
No regulation

Michigan
Board of Hearing Aid Dealers
Department of Licensing
  Regulation
P.O. Box 30018
Lansing, MI 48909
(517) 335-1699

Minnesota
Department of Health
717 S.E. Delaware Street
P.O. Box 9441
Minneapolis, MN 55440
(612) 623-5751

Missouri
Council for Hearing Aid
  Dealers and Fitters
P.O. Box 1335
Jefferson City, MO 65102
(314) 751-2334

Montana
Board of Hearing Aid
  Dispensers
Department of Professional and
  Occupational Licensing
1424 Ninth Avenue
Helena, MT 59601
(406) 444-3737

Nebraska
Board of Hearing Aid Dealers
  and Fitters
Bureau of Examining Boards
Department of Health
301 Centennial Mall South
P.O. Box 95007
Lincoln, NE 68509
(402) 471-2115

Nevada
State Board of Hearing Aid
  Specialists
1701 Lakeside Drive
Reno, NV 89509
(702) 322-3269

New Hampshire
Audiology and Hearing
  Instruments of New
  Hampshire
194 Pleasant Street, Suite 2A
Concord, NH 03301
(602) 224-3346
In state: 1 (800) 852-3783

New Jersey
State Board of Medical
  Examiners
28 West State Street
Trenton, NJ 08608
(609) 292-4843

New Mexico
Hearing Aid Advisory Board
P.O. Drawer 1388
Santa Fe, NM 87504-1388
(505) 827-4200

New York
Licensing Hearing Aid Dealers

Department of State
Division of Licensing Services
162 Washington Avenue
Albany, NY 12231
(518) 474-4664

North Carolina
Hearing Aid Dealers & Fitters
  Board
136 Oakwood Drive
Winston-Salem, NC 27103
(919) 722-0120

North Dakota
Hearing Aid Dealers and
  Fitters Board
Attorney General's Office
Licensing Division
State Capitol Building
Bismark, ND 58505
(701) 224-2219

Ohio
Hearing Aid Dealers Licensing
  Board
P.O. Box 118
Columbus, OH 43266
(614) 466-5215

Oklahoma
Hearing Aid Division
Occupational Licensing Service
Oklahoma State Health
  Department
P.O. Box 53551
Oklahoma City, OK 73152
(405) 271-5217

Oregon
Hearing Aid Licensing Board
P.O. Box 231

Portland, OR 97207
(503) 229-5780

Pennsylvania
Hearing Aid Dealers and Fitters
Department of Health
Division of Drugs, Devices and
  Cosmetics
P.O. Box 90
Health and Welfare Building,
  Room 930
Harrisburg, PA 17108
(717) 787-2307

Rhode Island
Bureau of Hearing Aid Dealers
  and Fitters
Department of Business
  Regulation
100 North Main Street
Providence, RI 02903
(401) 277-2416

South Carolina
Commission for Hearing Aid
  Dealers and Fitters
Department of Health and
  Environmental Control
Division of Health Licensing
2600 Bull Street
Columbia, SC 29201
(803) 734-4680

South Dakota
Board of Hearing Aid
  Dispensers
Department of Commerce
P.O. Box 1037
Pierre, SD 57501
(605) 224-1034

Tennessee
Board for Licensing Hearing
  Aid Dispensers

Department of Public Health
316 State Office Building
283 Plus Park Boulevard
Nashville, TN 37209-5407
(615) 387-6207

Texas
Board of Examiners for Fitting
and Dispensing of Hearing
Aids
4800 North Lamar, Suite 150
Austin, TX 78756
(512) 459-1488

Utah
Advisory Committee for
Hearing Aid Licensing
Department of Business
Regulation
160 East 300 South Street
P.O. Box 45802
Salt Lake City, UT 84145
(801) 530-6628

Vermont
Hearing Aid Dispenser
Secretary of State
Pavillion Office Building
Montpelier, VT 05602
(802) 828-2191

Virginia
Board of Hearing Aid Dealers
and Fitters

Department of Commerce
3600 West Broad Street
Richmond, VA 23230
(804) 367-8505

Washington
Department of Professional
Licensure–Hearing Aid
Dealers
P.O. Box 9649
Olympia, WA 98504
(208) 753-4616

West Virginia
Board of Hearing Aid Dealers
701 Jefferson Road
South Charleston, WV 25309
(304) 348-7886

Wisconsin
Hearing Aid Dealer and Fitter
Licensing Board
P.O. Box 8936
Madison, WI 53708
(608) 267-9377

Wyoming
Board of Hearing Aid
Specialists
5320 Education Drive
Cheyenne, WY 82009
(307) 635-0435

Index